Emma Newham's

BARRECONCEPT WORKOUT

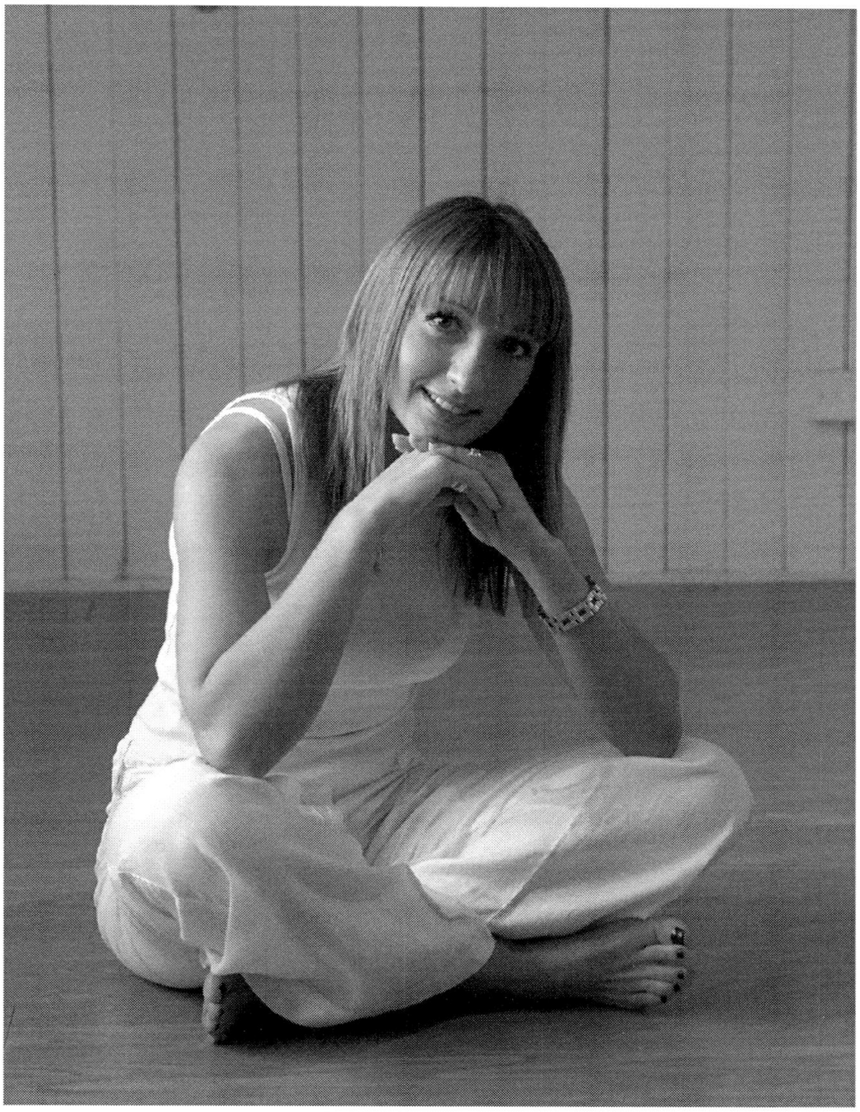

By Emma Newham

Published in the United Kingdom by

Pilates Union
MyBody Studios
Station Road
East Boldon
Tyne & Wear
NE36 0LE
www.pilatesunion.com

ISBN – 978-0-9565285-7-5

Emma Newham – Author

Printed in the UK by Jasprint

What is BarreConcept?

BarreConcept is a body sculpting method of exercise which combines the core strength, control and precision of Pilates with the positions, moves, grace and technique of ballet. Add to this the alignment of yoga and the strength from sports conditioning and you will have all of the aspects of a typical BarreConcept workout.

This regime has taken all of the best elements from each of the above methods to give a fantastic full body workout, which stretches and sculpts the muscles whilst burning fat, giving results that totally redefine the body. Balance, strength, stamina, power and motor control all improve.

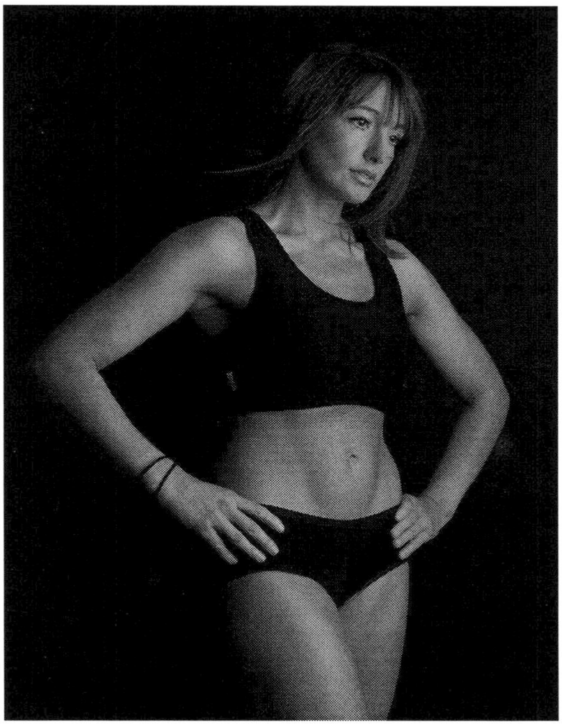

Workout Structure

Warm Up

The warm up is performed in the centre of the room, away from the barre. Movements including knee raises, tendus and small plies are performed to upbeat music in order to warm up the body, mobilise the joints and increase heart rate and cardiovascular efficiency. Arm movements should be included that reflect the basic five arm positions in ballet. Around five minutes is sufficient for the warm up.

Barre Work

The main bulk of the class (at least half of the lesson) should be spent at the barre. The main concentration of this section is focused on the legs and butt, although there are a few upper body exercises that may be performed here as well. In a traditional ballet class, the exercises performed at the barre are viewed as a preparation for the work done afterwards in the centre of the room. However, in a Barreconcept class, the work done at the barre is viewed as the main workout and so follows a different emphasis and structure.

In the Centre

Once the barre exercises have been completed, the workout then moves into the centre. This is where small, light hand weights may be included to work the upper body in terns of strength and endurance. Hand weight exercises are usually performed in conjunction with a leg movement in order to increase the heart rate and stamina.

Balance work should be included here as a progression from the work at the barre. Developpes, arabesques and penches as well as plies are performed in the centre.

Choreography should aim to string a series of movements together to contribute to the flow of the class. For example: - Pilie in first position, tendu to second position, plie in second position, tendu back to fifth position, Arabesque.

Power movements may be included at the end of the floorwork section such as ballet jumps in first or second in order to burn body fat and increase stamina. Less able clients or thos with knee problems should be offered an alternative such as releves (heel raises) instead.

Floor Work

Since there is limited upper body work and no abdominal exercises that can be done at the barre, this work is included in the floor work section. Leg and butt work may also be included in this section although less emphasis is needed for these muscle groups, since the majority of the exercises involving those muscle groups have been performed already at the barre. Since this is the lastcomponent of the class before the final stretch section, there is no need to stretch out the muscles following a particular exercise since it can wait until the end.

Final Stretches

Developmental stretches are performed at the end of the session, particularly for the legs and butt. Include stretches for the arms if upper body work has been executed during the floor work section. It is also prudent to mobilise and stretch the spinal muscles here since they are not generally performed at the barre or in the centre. This section should last up to five minutes.

Contractions, Repetitions, Static Holds and Sets

BarreConcept has a specific way of working the muscles in order to give maximum benefit and results.

Contractions

For certain exercises, a normal, full range concentric/ eccentric muscular contraction is performed. Other exercises involve a smaller range of concentric/ eccentric muscle contraction, usually performed at the end of a range of movement. Where stated, small isometric contractions are performed.

Repetitions

The number of repetitions performed for a given exercise is usually ten. These are generally performed slowly and with great control similar to the Pilates method.

Following the ten repetitions, certain exercises will involve twenty further repetitions, usually performed within a very small range of movement. Theses are generally performed right at the end of the range of movement with a pulsing type of muscular action similar to some sports conditioning techniques.

Following the twenty small pulses, certain exercises will then require a static hold similar to holding a yoga pose. Slow, deep yoga type breathing is done during the static hold. This final position is usually held for around ten seconds, although may be more/ less depending upon the ability of the client group.

Sets

A minimum of one set as performed above is required. Depending upon the needs and wants of the client group, up to two more sets may be done as necessary (e.g. if a particular muscle group needs to be targeted, then more sets of a particular exercise involving that muscle group may be performed).

The ability of the client group also needs to be taken into consideration. Some less able clients may not initially be able to perform the required repetitions, let alone the number of sets so this will need to be adapted and scaled down according to ability.

The other factor to take into account regarding the number of sets, is the amount of time it takes to complete them. Class planning and preparation needs to be considered, particularly if a lot of different exercises are to be fitted into the lesson plan. The more exercises to be fitted into the lesson, the less time there is available for the performance of sets.

Stretches

Short, static stretches are performed immediately following a muscular contraction and are held for around 10-30 seconds. This ensures that the fatigued muscles are re-lengthened straight away to prevent any muscle shortening and to minimise stiffness and fatigue. Stretches are therefore done throughout the class. In addition, some developmental stretches for the larger muscle groups may also chosen to be performed at the end of the class.

A typical exercise will therefore be performed as follows:-

10 x slow repetitions

20 x small pulses

10 second static hold

Another set if required

Immediate stretch for the muscle group being contracted

Basic Workout Principles

Since BarreConcept contains elements of Pilates, we will refer to some of the basic positions and principles as found below.

Pelvic Positions

Aim

To find the natural curve of the lumbar spine so that we can learn correct placement of the spine for future exercises

Starting Position

Lie supine on your back on the floor with the knees bent and the feet flat on the floor, hip distance apart. A small head cushion may be placed underneath the skull in order to place the cervical spine in its natural position.

Action

Finding the North Position of the Pelvis

Inhale to prepare. As you exhale, gently tilt the pelvis backwards into a posterior tilt. The pubic bone will point up to the ceiling. The pubic bone will be higher than the hipbones resulting in the lumbar spine being lengthened towards flexion. The lower back will press down into the floor.

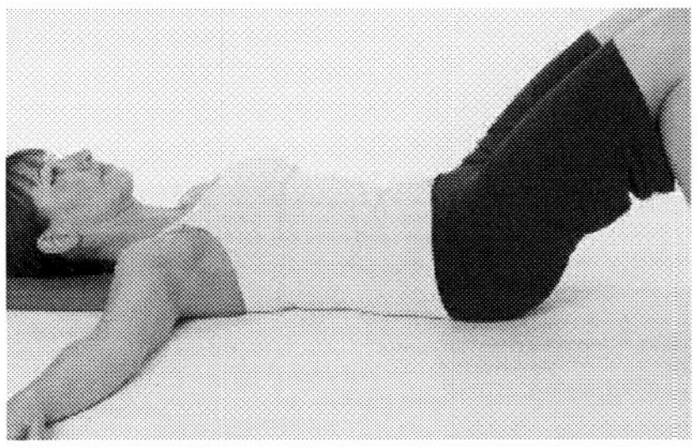

North pelvic position

Finding the South Position of the Pelvis

Inhale to prepare. As you exhale, gently tilt the pelvis forwards into an anterior tilt. The pubic bone will point down to the floor. The hipbones will now be higher than the pubic bone, resulting in the lumbar spine being in an extended position. The lower back will arch away from the floor.

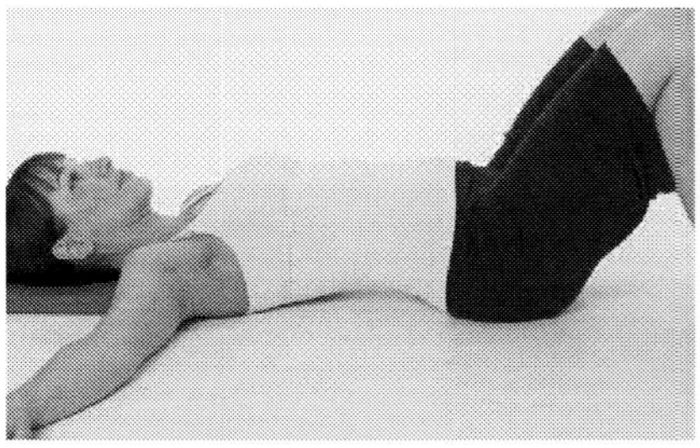

South pelvic position

Finding the Neutral Position of the Pelvis

Tilt the pelvis gently north, then centre and then south and return to the centre a few times and come to rest half way between the two points. The true definition of a neutral pelvis is when the anterior superior iliac spine (ASIS) is level with the pubic symphysis (i.e. if you got a spirit level between each hip bone and the pubic bone, all bones would be level at the same plane and height). Ideally this neutral pelvis should feel natural but because of different postural types, this may not be the case. A neutral position should not be forced if it feels uncomfortable in any way. If it does not happen naturally initially, then it is something to work towards as the body gets stronger.

Watchpoints

- Try not to grip in the hip flexors and glutes.
- Maintain good alignment with the hip, knee and second toe.
- Ensure that the back of the neck stays long and the shoulders stay away from the ears.

Pelvic Stability

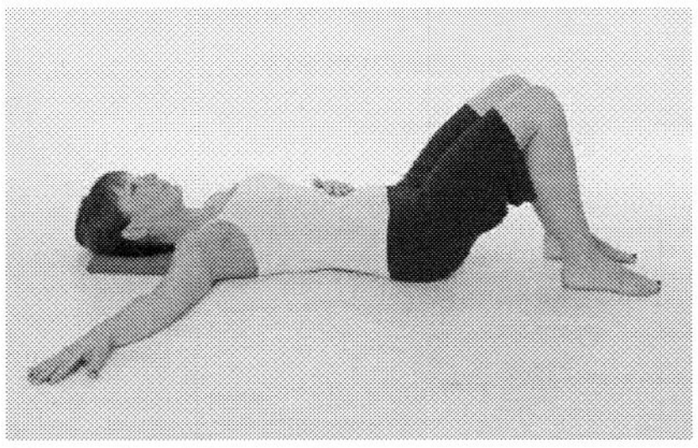

Neutral pelvic position

The combination of the transversus abdominis, a deep back muscle known as the multifidus and also the pelvic floor muscles make up our core. The correct engagement of these core muscles will hold our pelvis in the safe neutral position whilst we are performing our exercises. This helps to prevent any tilting or arching of the lumbar spine, causing potential stress to the lower back. We call this pelvic stability.

Transversus Abdominis

We shall learn how to engage the transversus abdominus in 4 different positions. Remember we only need to recruit this muscle by about 30%. The reasons that we recruit at a low level is that we need to try to isolate these muscles in order to prevent other stronger muscles helping out and doing the job of the core. Also, the core muscles should be working for the whole of our Pilates class and if they are engaged too much then they will fatigue very quickly. We need them for endurance so a low level of recruitment will make them last longer. "Less is more" – the less you contract, the more you will be able to isolate. The harder you contract, the less you will be able to isolate.

Position One – Relaxation Position

Starting Position

Lie supine in the relaxation position with the knees bent and the feet hip distance apart. A small head cushion may be placed underneath the skull in order to place the cervical spine in its natural position. Find the neutral position of the pelvis. You may like to slide the fingertips of one hand underneath the natural lumbar curve in order to check that the pelvis remains in a neutral position. Ensure that the body does not move an inch as you slide the fingertips under. Check that there is an even pressure on the fingers throughout the exercise (i.e. no decrease in pressure if the pelvis tilts south and no increase in pressure if the pelvis tilts north). You may place the opposite hand on top of the belly.

Action

Inhale to prepare. Exhale and gently draw in the navel back down towards the spine. Try to achieve around 30% contraction. If you are unsure what 30% feels like then contact the navel as hard as you can (i.e. 100%). Then release the contraction by half (i.e. 50%). Then release by half again and that will be around 25% contraction.

Watchpoints

- Watch out for any tension in the body, particularly around the neck and shoulders
- Keep the length between ears and shoulders and the back of the neck long
- Ensure that there is not change in pressure on the hand that is under the pelvis as you engage the transversus abdominus
- Try not to grip around the hip flexors, buttocks or legs

Position Two – Lying Prone

Starting Position

Lie face down on the floor with the legs together. The elbows are bent and the hands rest under the forehead, palms facing down.

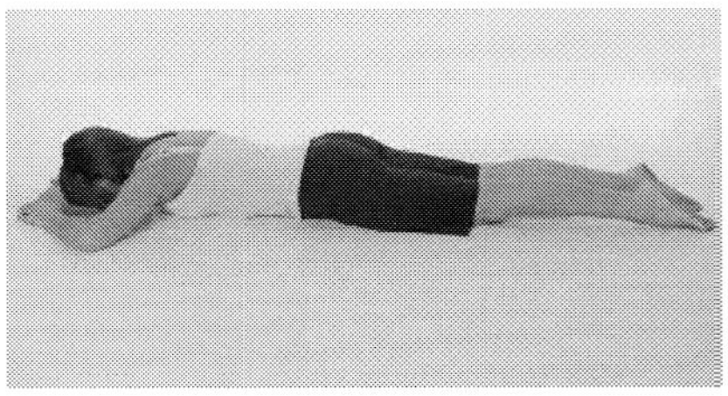

Action

As you inhale, imagine the abdomen and waistline are expanding, almost like a balloon filling with air. Exhale and pull the navel in back towards the spine against gravity. Imagine you have a precious egg underneath the abdomen and you are gently taking the pressure off it. You could almost slide a piece of paper under the belly.

Watchpoints

- As you pull in the navel ensure that the buttocks do not engage or the pelvis move
- Maintain the distance between ears and shoulders

Contra-Indications

If lying prone feels uncomfortable initially for certain back problems, then place a small cushion underneath the hipbones.

Position Three – Kneeling on all fours

Starting Position

Come to an all fours position with the knees bent directly under the hips and place the hands on the floor directly under the shoulders. The elbows are soft and the fingers are pointing forwards. Ensure that there is equal weight between the hands and feet and between right and left sides of the body by gently rocking the body forward and back and from side to side a little. Allow the body weight to come to rest between all four limbs equally. Keep a good length between the ears and shoulders. The back of the neck should follow the natural cervical curves.

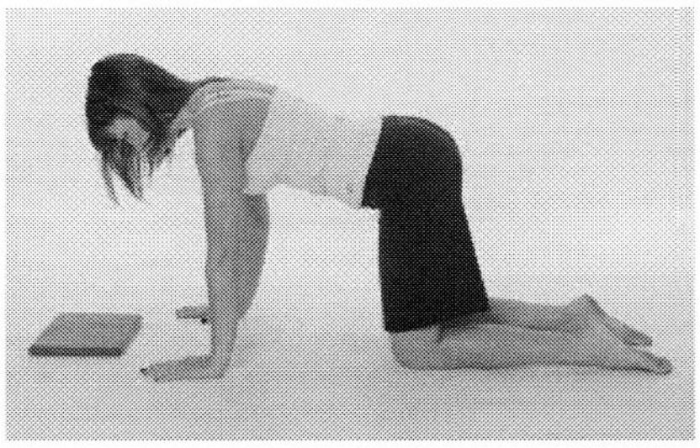

Action

Find the neutral pelvis by tilting the pelvis north and south and coming to rest half way in between. Inhale to prepare. As you exhale, gently pull in the navel back towards the spine against gravity. Imagine there is a scalding hot cup of tea balancing on the pelvis and lumbar spine so that as the navel is pulled in, the tea does not spill.

Watchpoints

- As the navel is pulled in, ensure that the back does not arch
- Maintain the gap between the ears and the shoulders
- Do not allow the shoulder blades to collapse together. Pull the shoulder blades apart on the ribcage using the serratus anterior muscle.
- There is a tendency for the head to start to drop downwards. Ensure that the back of the neck stays long with the back of the skull pushing up towards the ceiling.
- Ensure that the elbows do not lock out as the joint should stay soft

Contra-Indications

This position places extra stress on the wrist and knee joints and may be unsuitable for clients with problems in these joints.

Pelvic Floor

Most people have a vague idea of where the pelvic floor muscles are located and what they do but they may not be aware of all of the different openings from front to back. These are the muscles that stop us from "going to the toilet". Women have three openings and men have two. You will be shown how to isolate each opening of the pelvic floor separately in order to be familiar with each section. Then, when each component part has been felt, you can engage the entire area as one whole.

Together with the transversus abdominus muscle, the pelvic floor forms what we refer to as the "core", so they are very important.

When we are learning to isolate each opening, the amount of contraction is very small indeed. This is because the openings are very close together and if you engage one opening too much, the other openings will also contract.

It is impossible to tell if somebody is performing pelvic floor correctly, since no movement in the body can be detected. However, you can tell if somebody is doing it incorrectly, since external movement can be seen. Common mistakes include gripping in the glutes and hip flexors or tilting the pelvis or tensing the legs.

It is not always obvious when you engage the contraction, whether you have managed to isolate a particular opening or not. It is more obvious as the contraction is released. You may think to yourself "Ah, I felt my buttocks relax there". In which case, the glutes have engaged as well as the pelvic floor but you may not have realised that when you contracted the muscles. So, it is easier to tell when you let go of the contraction, since you will sense other parts also release. If this is the case, then remember, "Less is more". The less you contract, the more you will be able to isolate. So next time, contract a little less. These kegel exercises are best done with the eyes closed. With the eyes open, the brain tends to take in visual stimulus from around the room. When the eyes are closed, the brain is free to concentrate on the internal environment and becomes more sensitive to different sensations within the body (i.e. you can "feel"more).

The relaxation position is the preferred position in which to practice pelvic floor contractions although it may be done in any position such as side lying, sitting upright, standing or on all fours. The relaxation position has been chosen since it is a comfortable position within which to work as the body is relaxed and the mind therefore free to concentrate.

Pelvic floor isolation - Starting Position

Lie supine in the relaxation position with the knees bent and the feet flat on the floor, hip distance apart. A small head cushion may be placed underneath the skull in order to place the cervical spine in its natural position. You may like to slide the fingertips of one hand underneath the natural lumbar curve in order to check that the pelvis remains in a neutral position.

The back passage opening – The sphincter muscle

Action

Inhale to prepare. As you exhale, gently and slowly start to contract your back passage (your bottom hole) by drawing it inwards and upwards. This is your sphincter muscle and the sensation you want to achieve is that you are stopping yourself from passing wind. It is very tempting to squeeze the cheeks of the bottom here so be aware. Hold the contraction for around 5 seconds, continuing to exhale as you hold the contraction. Then inhale to release the contraction and see if you are able to tell if you managed to isolate the sphincter muscle.

The front passage opening –

Action

Inhale to prepare. As you exhale, gently and slowly start to contract the front passage (this is the muscle that you pee out of) by drawing it inwards and upwards. The sensation you need to achieve here is that you are stopping or lessening the flow of urine mid flow. Try not to grip around the hip flexors or legs here and ensure that the pelvis does not tilt. Hold the contraction for 5 seconds whilst exhaling and inhale to release and see if you were able to isolate again.

The middle passage – The vagina (women only!!)

Action

Inhale to prepare. As you exhale slowly and gently contract the walls of the vagina by drawing the muscle inwards and upwards. Imagine an elevator in your mind. Visualise the elevator doors closing. The walls of the vagina have to come together in a similar way, almost like drawing a pair of curtains together. You may also like to imagine a drawstring bag or purse. When the string is pulled, the gap tightens together. Then the walls of the vagina need to lift upwards to the first floor (towards the navel) and then continue lifting up to the second floor (towards the ribs). So the action is to draw the curtains first and then lift up to the various floors after. Hold the contraction for 5 seconds whilst exhaling and inhale to release and see if you were able to isolate again.

Men only!!

In addition to the front and back passage, it may be helpful to feel like you are lifting up "the family jewels".

Neutral Spine

So far, you have learned that the combination of the transversus abdominus and pelvic floor muscles stabilise the lumbar spine and pelvis into a neutral position. This is important when there is a leg movement involved, which can potentially pull on the lower back. In addition, the oblique muscles prevent the ribcage from flaring out, thereby pulling the upper back out of a neutral position, particularly when there is an arm movement involved. This next exercise involves sliding the leg and opposite arm away from the body. Therefore you will need to engage all three areas in order to stabilise the entire spine (not just the pelvis or upper back on their own) into a neutral position. The three areas should be engaged in the following order; pelvic floor, transversus abdominus and obiques.

Here, you will have the weight of two limbs potentially pulling the spine out of a neutral position. However, t is not necessarily the weight of the limbs that will make the back arch – it is the brain instead! When learning a new skill, the brain tends to focus on one thing at a time. Up until now, it has only had one limb to contend with and it was therefore easier to move a single limb whilst holding onto the core muscles. Now the brain has two limbs to think about, so the element of co-ordination has entered into the equation. The brain now has the breathing, the core engagement and the co-ordination of opposite limbs to negotiate. Initially, it is unlikely that all these elements will be correctly activated at once. For example, you may have perfect breathing and perfect co-ordination but the pelvic floor may be relaxed. If any part of the core abdominals is not engaged, then you are not practicing safe and effective technique and not doing Pilates correctly. Don't worry initially if your co-ordination is poor or if the breathing is not quite right. It is more important to have the core engaged correctly over the co-ordination or breathing since the back is vulnerable to stress if these muscles are not working properly. Get the core right first and then the breathing and co-ordination will follow.

Starfish

To learn how to maintain a neutral spine, whilst moving two limbs away from the body

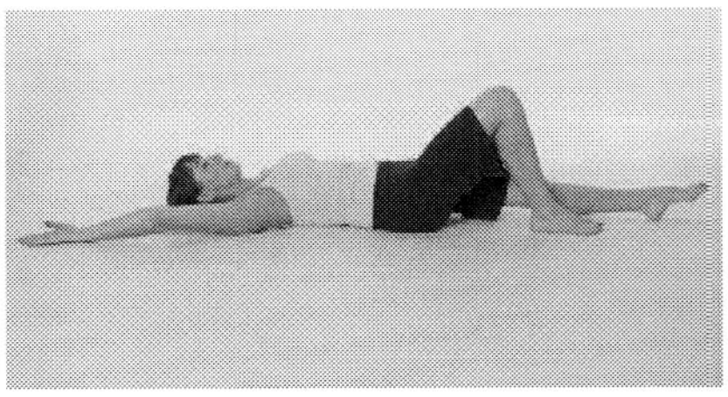

Starting Position

Lie supine in the relaxation position with the knees bent and the feet flat on the floor, hip distance apart. A small head cushion may be placed underneath the skull in order to place the cervical spine in its natural position. The arms are down by the sides of the body.

Action

Inhale to prepare. Exhale engage the pelvic floor openings first, followed by the transversus abdominus and finally the obliques. It is almost like pulling up a zip on your jeans. Start low with the pelvic floor and work your way up to the transverses, then draw down the ribcage. Once these core muscles are correctly engaged, continue exhaling and gently slide one leg along the floor, away from the body until it is straight. Simultaneously raise the opposite arm upwards to the ceiling and overhead as far as flexibility allows, without forcing the arm back. Inhale, continuing to keep the abdominals engaged and gently use the core muscles to bend the knee and draw the leg and arm back in towards the body.

Watchpoints

Only push the arm and leg as far as a neutral spine allows

The collar bones should be wide, the neck long and the shoulders away from the ears

Do not force the arm back, stay within a good range of movement so as not to compromise technique

Ensure that the shoulder, elbow and wrist stay in alignment (don't bend the elbow or flick the wrist)

Opposition

This is the principle of lengthening whilst strengthening. Think of energy lines in the body and try to push the limbs in opposing directions along these lines, whilst maintaining a strong centre. In order to experience this, try the following exercise firstly without opposition and then using opposition.

Lie on your side with the arm outstretched and the head resting on the shoulder. The underneath leg is bent forwards and the top leg is outstretched straight along the floor in alignment with the spine. Relax the body and do not stretch the leg. Perform the exercise in a lazy way in order to feel the difference between the two methods. Just raise the top leg up off the floor a few inches until the foot is just above hip height. Ask yourself two questions. "Where do you feel the muscle contraction?' and "How intense is the workload?". Give it a mark out of 10 for effort (1 being minimal, easy effort and 10 being hard, maximal effort). The answer to the first question should be; outer thigh. The workload is usually fairly low, generally below 5 out of 10 depending upon ability. Now try the same exercise using opposition.

Lie on your side with the arm outstretched and the head resting on the shoulder. Walk the fingers of this hand along the floor so that the arm is really lengthening. Feel energy coming out of the crown of the head, almost like the head is being pulled by a piece of string attached to it, so that it too lengthens along the arm. Think of the 3 body spaces. The gap between the ear and shoulder is wide. Also the gap between the last rib and the iliac crest (i.e. the waist) is long. Finally, make space in the hip joint (i.e. lengthen the femur out of the hip socket). The top arm is bent in front of the body and the hand is pressing downwards into the floor whilst the elbow is reaching upwards to the ceiling in opposition.

The underneath leg is bent forwards and the top leg is outstretched straight along the floor in alignment with the spine. Lengthen the toes of the top leg along the floor to achieve a long leg. Pull up the knee-cap so that the thighs are firm. The whole body from the fingers to the toes should now be long. Imagine that your body is on an old fashioned rack, being pulled apart in two different directions. The head and underneath arm are lengthening northwards, whilst the waist and top leg are lengthening southwards. Watch you don't buckle in the middle!! A strong centre is needed to prevent the spine from arching. Make good use of the full powerhouse here in order to keep a neutral spine whilst lengthening.

Raise the leg as before but don't just lift and lower the leg, keep lengthening it the whole time.

Now ask yourself the same two questions. The answer to question one should still be "outer thigh" but in addition, the whole body is involved. Before, the rest of the body may have been relaxed and so the effort was just felt in one area. With opposition, the outer thigh is the primary muscle working but the whole body is lengthening and working as well in order to maintain the length. The intensity should therefore be well above a 5 out of 10 now. See how much effort lengthening the body involves? It takes a lot of energy to work in this way. The results, however, speak for themselves. It is the length rather than any height in the leg that makes this exercise (or any exercise for that matter) much harder. This sets Pilates apart from a normal body conditioning class. It is "how" you do it. Quality of movement over quantity, or number of repetitions. Try the Star exercise where all four limbs are stretched out. Here, you have 4 energy lines pulling in 4 opposing directions. The right arm is reaching forwards to the right hand corner of the room whilst the left arm is reaching forwards to the left hand corner of the room. In addition the right leg is reaching backwards to the back right hand corner of the room, whilst the left leg is reaching backwards to the back left hand corner of the room. Whenever you are working, keep thinking about the energy lines in the body and try to create as much length as possible, whilst keeping a strong centre

BarreConcept Workout format

What follows are pages of the typical exercises that are used in a BarreConcept class. Beginners should learn each exercise in isolation initially in order to grasp correct technique and good movement patterns. However, the aim is to join several exercise moves together to form a flowing, choreographed routine, without a break.

Below is a typical BarreConcept class example. It is impossible to include every exercise featured in this manual in one class, so there are many variations on this theme. It will, however, give you an idea of how to format a workout routine. This may be adapted and changed where necessary in order to cater for different needs and capabilities.

Warm Up

a) Legs in parallel and hip width apart. Relevé onto demi pointe and raise the arms up to fifth position. Lower the heels under resistance and bring the arms to first position x 8.
b) Plié in parallel and raise arms to fifth position as the knees bend x 8.
c) Hold the plié in parallel and raise the arms up and down from fifth to first x 8 (this may be done on demi pointe)
d) Hold the plié and raise and lower the heels x 8
e) Plié in second position x 8 full range.
f) Plié into tendu on right leg x 8. Repeat to left x 8. Repeat alternating legs x 8
g) Plié into curtsey behind (right leg crosses behind) x 4. Repeat to left x 4. Repeat alternating legs x 8
h) Plié into side leg abduction and arms raise out to opposite direction x 8 on right side. Repeat to left x 8
i) Plié into side bend to right x 8. Repeat to left x 8.
j) Alternate knee lifts forward x 8. Alternate knee lifts out to side x 8.
k) Alternate leg kicks forward x 8
l) Plié in second then turn torso to the right, bringing both legs into a lunge with both knees bent at 90 degrees. Raise the front heel so that both heels are off the floor (the back heel is already off the floor). Pulse up and down a few inches within the lunge position, maintaining the demi pointe x 8. Repeat to the left x 8.

Barre Work

a) **1.** Stand sideways to barre. Relevé onto demi pointe. Plié in parallel x 4 repetitions in full range of motion. Hold plié and pulse (mini mid range movements) up and down an inch x 8. Repeat twice if desired.

2. Relevé onto demi pointe in parallel and plié. Hold the plié and perform 4 x slow followed by 8 x quick Pelvic Tilts (north to neutral).

b) **1.** Turn to face the opposite direction. Plié in first position x 4 slow repetitions in full range of motion. Hold plié and pulse up and down an inch x 8. This may be done on demi pointe. Repeat twice if desired.

2. Relevé onto demi point in first position and plié. Hold the plié, then close and open the knees, performing 4 x slow and then 8 x quick Inner Thigh Squeezes.

3. On demi pointe, alternate performing one inner thigh squeeze followed by one pelvic tilt x 8 of each.

c) Plié in second and lift right heel x 4. Repeat with the left heel x 4. Alternate lifting each heel (i.e. as one heel raises, the other heel lowers and vice versa) x 8. Then raise and lower both heels x 8. Perform a standing Quadriceps stretch..

d) **1**. Plié in second and side bend towards the barre. Simultaneously turn the body to face the barre, bringing both legs into a 90 degree angle lunge and back to plié again x 8.

2. Back lunge. Standing upright facing the barre, lift the right knee up to the chest and then bend both knees, leaning away from the barre, extending the right leg backwards into a lunge and then straighten the left leg and bring the right knee into the chest again x 8. The right foot, however, does not touch the floor on the back lunge and the hands remain on the barre throughout. Then hold the lunge position with the right foot off the floor for a count of 8.

3. Hamstring Press. Standing upright facing the barre, bend the right knee, bringing the heel towards the butt until a 90 degree angle at the knee is held (ankle level to knee). Slightly bend the supporting left knee and hold this position whilst pushing the right leg back behind the body (maintaining the 90 degree angle). The sole of the foot faces away as the leg pulses back x 4 slow followed by 8 x quick repetitions.

4. Oyster. Both knees are bent (as for exercise 3 above). Bend both elbows out to the side and rest them on the barre with the forehead placed on the hands. Open out the right leg to the side, maintaining the 90 degree angle at the knee x 4 slow then x 8 quick pulses. Then circle the leg forwards x 4 and backwards x 4.

Repeat the above sequence (exercise 1-3) on the opposite side. Perform a standing Quadriceps stretch, Hamstring stretch on the barre and standing Glute stretch.

e) Press Ups facing the barre. 8 x double count (i.e. 2 counts to bend the elbows and 2 counts to straighten). 8 x single counts. Repeat twice.

Single arm press ups x 8 on each side.

Barre Work cont'd

f) **1.** Superman exercise facing the barre with the torso parallel to the floor. Lift and lower one leg in full range of motion from the floor to hip height x 8. Then hold the leg up at hip height and pulse the leg up and down an inch x 8. Hold the leg at hip height and pulse the leg out to the side in abduction an inch x 8. Pulse the leg inwards in adduction an inch x 8.

2. Hamstring Curls in superman position. Hold the leg straight out at hip height and bend the knee, bringing the heel towards the butt. Ensure the knee does not drop below hip height x 8. (This may also be performed standing with the torso upright).

3. Glute Press. Hold the hamstring curl position above with the knee at hip height, bent at 90 degrees. Lift the leg upwards an inch or two, with the sole of the foot facing the ceiling (maintain the 90 degree angle) x 8.

Repeat with the left leg. Perform a standing hamstring stretch and a glute stretch as before.

g) Standing upright, facing the barre, curtsey the right leg behind the left and then abduct the right leg out to the side x 8. Repeat with the left leg.

h) Stand sideways onto the barre and plié in first then relevé onto demi pointe (maintaining the plié), straighten both legs and then lower the heels to the floor x 8. Repeat the sequence in second position turning to face the opposite direction.

i) **1.** Stand sideways on to the barre. Plié in second and come to retiré, then plié second again and close into first x 4. This may also be performed on demi pointe when coming to retiré. This may also be done with a sauté from first to second to add some power work into the routine.

2. Plié in second and raise the outside leg into grand battement to the side, then plié in second and lift the leg into attitude x 4

3. Lunge backwards with the outside leg, keeping the back leg straight with the ball of the foot on the floor and then raise the back leg up to retiré x 8 (may also be done on demi pointe).

Repeat the above sequence facing the opposite direction.

j) Side Kick Karate x 8 on each side.

k) Facing away with back against the barre and arms outstretched along the barre – Grand Battements. Alternate between lifting right and left leg. Then perform attitude to the front alternating sides each time.

l) Mermaid Stretch. Standing hip flexor stretch. Standing glute stretch. Spinal rotation stretch.

In the Centre

a) Plié in second position, whilst performing, The Waiter. As the knees bend, the arms open. Straighten the legs to return the arms to the starting position x 8

b) Front Lunge with the front knee bent and the back leg straight. Perform The Chariot x 8. Then change legs to perform Tricep extension with both arms

c) Low arabesque position (foot just a few inches off floor if possible with the leg in parallel). Perform a front shoulder raise as the back leg raises a few inches. As the arms lower, the leg lowers (but ideally does not touch the floor) x 8 on each leg. The supporting knee is slightly bent.

d) Battement tendu front whilst performing a Chest Press x 4, followed by an overhead press x 4. Then alternate 1 x chest press with 1 x overhead press (4 of each).

e) Standing side leg abduction with lateral shoulder raise x 4 on the right leg. Repeat with the left x 4. Then do 8 x alternate lifts.

f) Plié in second position and transfer to an arabesque on the right leg. Simultaneously perform The Aeroplane. Repeat to the left. Alternate x 4 each side.

g) Ballet Jumps or elevés as a modification. (This may also be performed at the barre).

   1. Jumps in First x 8.
   2. Jumps in Second x 8.
   3. Jumps from First to Second x 8.
   4. Changements x 8.

Floor Work

a) **1.** Lean backs with arm release. Roll back with hands behind the knees and release right arm off in the air and hold for a count of 8. Roll back up. Repeat with the left arm x 8 counts. Roll back up. Repeat with both arms in the air x 8. Then lift and lower the arms from first to fifth x 8, whilst holding the lean back. Roll up.

   2. Lean back with oblique twist. Roll back and release the right arm off in the air and oblique twist to the left x 8 counts. Then perform small oblique pulses to the left x 8. Roll up. Repeat with the left arm in the air x 8 counts. Then perform small oblique pulses to the right x 8. Roll back up.

   3. Pelvic tilts in lean back position x 8. Roll up.

b) Oblique curl ups (one leg straight, one leg bent) x 8 slow followed by 8 x quick pulse to each side.

c) Scissors x 8 on each leg.

d) Diamond leg lowers x 8.

e) Quadricep lean backs x 8 plus pelvic rocks x 8

f) Mermaid in attitude x 8 on each leg plus 8 x pulses

g) Side lying developpé x 8 on each leg

h) Plank position with knee bend variations x 16 alternate knee bends.

i) ¾ Press Ups x 8 slow. Hold for a count of 8. 8 x mid range pulses.

j) Stretches – Quads, Hamstrings, Hip Flexor, Glutes, Adductors, Mermaid.

THE EXERCISES

WARM UP

AT THE BARRE

IN THE CENTRE

FLOOR WORK

THE STRETCHES

WARM UP

A BarreConcept warm up lasts around five minutes. It is designed to increase body temperature and mobilise the major joints so ensure knee lifts, straight leg kicks and pliés are included. Small preparatory movements which will later be used later in the class are included here. The barrework may also be considered a warm up for work done in the centre of the room afterwards. Below is an example of some typical movements used in the warm up. The warm up should be performed at a brisk pace to up tempo music. For a description of the full warm up typical format, see the pages BarreConcept Workout Format – Warm up.

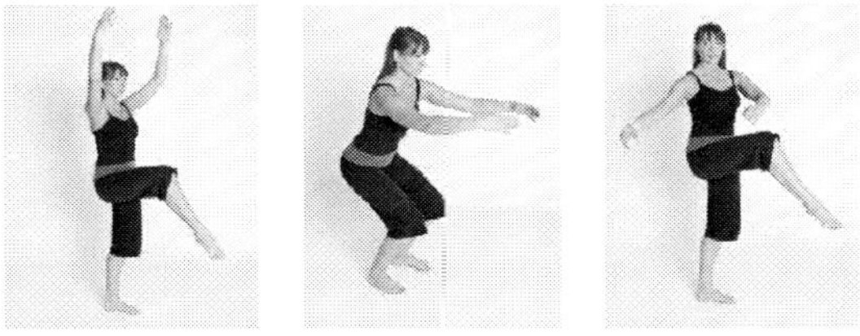

Squat down (arms up) and lift right knee (arms down). Repeat left knee. Alternating knee lifts (no squat).

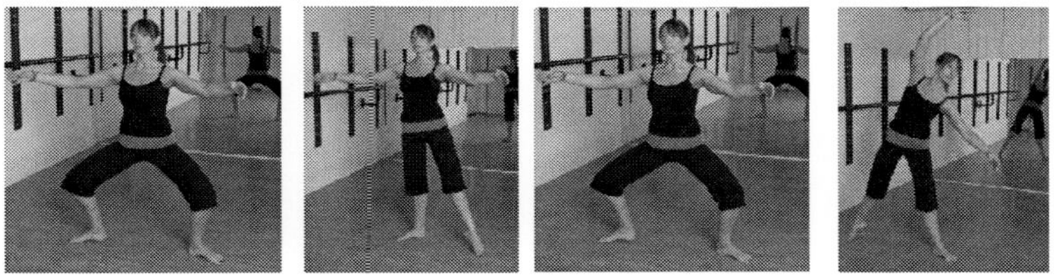

Plié in Second position and point alternate feet (transfer weight in between). Plié and side bend over to the right. Repeat to left. Alternate sides.

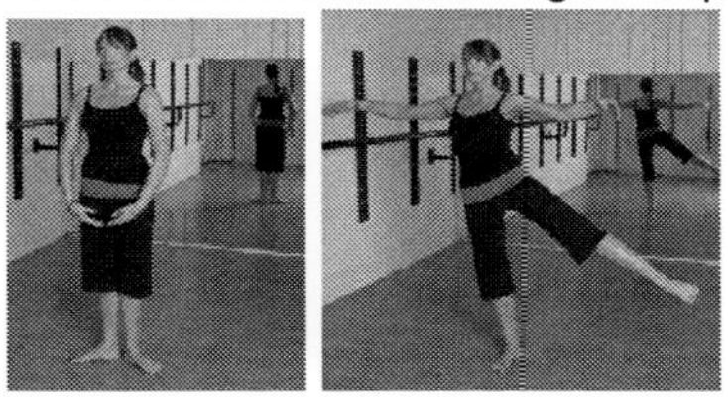

Plié and right leg abducts. Repeat to left. Full circumduction with arms

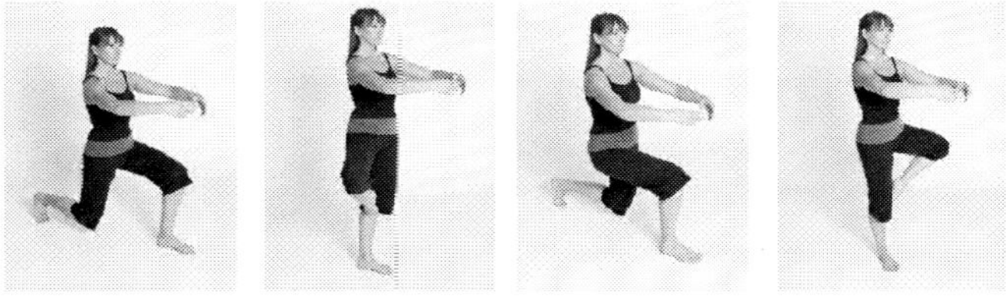

Front lunge into retiré Back lunge into retiré on each leg

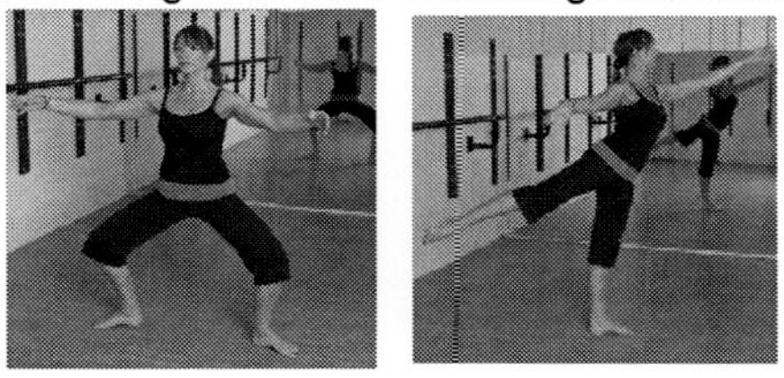

Plié in Second position into arabesque. Then hold arabesque and pulse leg

AT THE BARRE

Glossary of Ballet Terms
Basic Ballet Positions
Battements Tendu
Battements Glissé (Degagé)
Grand Battements
Plié Series
Fondue
Elevé
Relevés
Inner Thigh Squeeze
Pelvic Tilts
Developpés
Attitude
Hamstring Curl
Superman
Leg Abduction Series
Quadricep Lifts
Press Ups
Pull Ups
V Stretch against the Wall
Handstand Preparation One
Handstand Preparation Two
Mermaid Stretch
Hamstring Stretch Variations
Side Splits
Swan Stretch
Standing Glute Stretch
Stabding Quad Stretch
Standing Hip Flexor Stretch
Standing Spinal Twist

Glossary of Terms used in BarreConcept

A la Seconde – Second Position or to the side

A Terre – On the ground

Attitude – A ballet position standing on one leg whilst the other leg is lifted back with the knee bent at 90 degrees and turned out so that the knee is higher than the foot. The arm on the same side as the raised leg is held above the head (as in Fifth position) whilst the other arm is extended out to the side (unless on the barre).

Battement – To beat or kick. Battements may be performed to the front, side or back.
Petit Battements - refer to tendus, frappes, degagés, glissés and relevés
Grand Battements - A powerful action, where the leg is kicked in the air with ease, as high as possible, whilst the supporting leg and torso remain stable and straight. The accent is on the downward movement.

Croisé – Crossed

Degagé – To disengage. This is similar to tendu except that the foot leaves the floor (anywhere from an inch to 45 degrees but usually around 4 inches off the floor). It is done at twice the speed as a tendu. This exercise strengthens the toes, improves mobility of the ankle joint and develops the instep

Demi – Half. Demi pointe is a position of the feet where the heels are raised off the floor onto the balls of the feet. Demi plié is a half knee bend.
Derrieré - Behind

Devant – In front

Developpé - To develop. The working leg is drawn up to the knee of the supporting leg and then unfolds, extending to either the front, side or back in the air (en l'air) with control, maintaining pelvic stability.

Elevé and Relevé – To rise. Rising up onto pointe or demi-pointe from flat feet onto the balls of the feet. Elevé is a relevé without the plié

En Dehors – Clockwise direction (outwards)

En Dedans – Anticlockwise direction (inwards)

En l' air – In the air

Fondu – To melt. A bending of one knee to lower the body (single leg Plié)

Glissé – To glide. This is the same step as degage

Plié – To bend. Basically a knee bend which may be performed as a demi plié (half bend) or a grand plié (full bend until the thighs are horizontal). The heels remain on the floor in a demi plié but they raise off the floor for the grand plié (except for the open positions of Second and Fourth where the heels remain on the floor). though they should remain on the floor for as long as possible when performing the grand plié). This exercise can be done at the barre or in the centre in all five basic positions (although not usually done in Third position).

Retiré – To withdraw. Raise one leg out to second position in the air (en l'air) and bend the knee so that the pointed toe rests either in front, behind or to the side of the supporting knee

Ronds de jambe – Round of the leg. This refers to the circular movement made by the working leg and may be done at the barre or in the centre and may be performed in a clockwise or anticlockwise direction.
Rond de jambe a terre is performed on the ground. Both legs remain straight and the movement of the working leg comes from the hip. The toe remains on the floor and does not pass beyond Fourth position in front or behind. The heel should remain forwards and the toe back.
Rond de jambe en l'air is performed in the air and may be performed as a single or double action. The working leg is held out in Second position in the air. The thigh is kept horizontal whilst all the movement occurs below the knee. A circular oval motion is made when the pointed toe of the working foot brushes the inside of the supporting knee before the leg is once again extended.

Sauté – To jump

Sickle – A faulty winging position of the foot that breaks the line of the leg. The foot inverts towards the body instead of away thereby losing alignment of the leg and foot.

Tendu – To stretch. The working leg slides away from First or Fifth position to Second or Fourth position without leaving the floor. The legs are straight and the heel leaves the floor but the toe does not and the instep is stretched. Once the position has been reached, it then returns to the original starting position.

Turn-out
Classical ballet is performed with a turned out stance. This position refers to the external rotation of the legs from the hip socket. This results in the knees and feet turning outwards, away from the body. The ankles remain stable and the arch of the foot maintains its supporting curve. Not everybody can turnout well and this must not be forced. Improper turnout will result in the knee pointing forwards whilst the foot points out to the side (i.e. turning out from the knee instead of the hip) and the ankle will roll inwards, placing stress on the knee and ankle joint.

Five Basic Ballet Positions of the arms and feet

Bras Bas

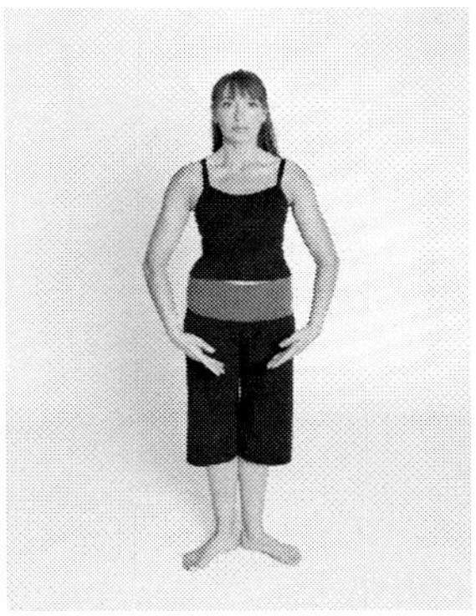

Arms are low and down. The arms are held down in front of the body in a soft circular arc shape, with the palms facing each other elbows soft and fingers soft and long. The back edge of the hands (but not the elbows) rests on the thighs. This is almost a rest position and is used as a starting or preparatory position for many exercises.

First Position

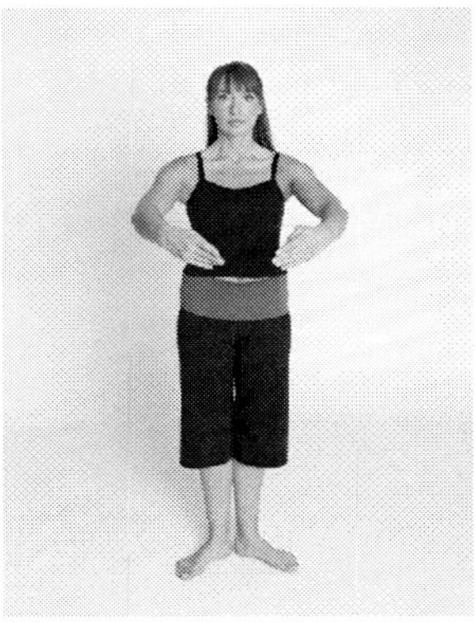

Legs – Stand in a parallel stance with the knees and feet together. Externally rotate the legs out from the hip socket resulting in the heels being together and the toes apart. This is the basic turn out position. Ideally the feet form one line.
Arms - The arms are held in front of the body below shoulder height. The elbows are soft and the arms form a soft arc shape (like hugging a tree). The spine and neck are long and the shoulders relaxed. The fingers are soft yet long and not quite touching each other.

Second Position

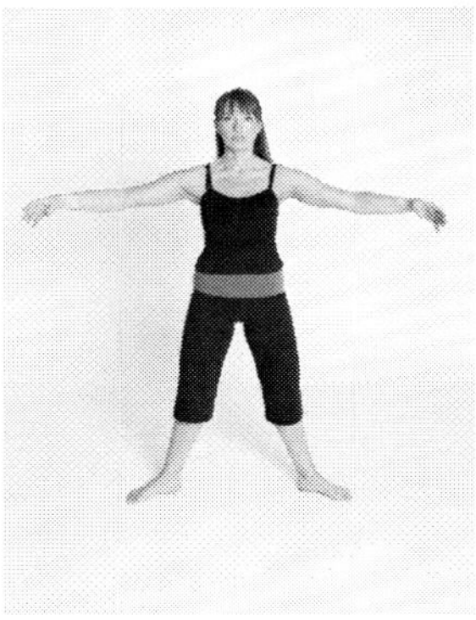

Legs – From First position, the feet are on the same line but with a distance of about one foot between the heels.
Arms – From First position, open out the arms laterally, maintaining the elbows below shoulder height. The elbows are soft and the arms form a wide arc shape. The wrists are lower than the elbows. The spine and neck are long.

Third Position

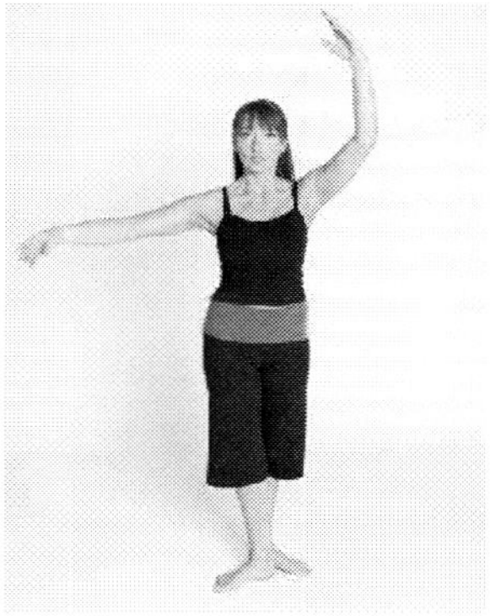

Legs - The legs are externally rotated out from the hip socket as in First position. However, in this instance, one leg is crossed directly in front of the other with the heel of the front foot touching the middle of the foot that is behind

Arms – The arms work in opposition to the legs (i.e. the left arm is raised if the right foot is in front). Raise the left arm up (not directly above the head but slightly in front) whilst opening out the right arm to the side (similar to Second position) and level to the navel.

Fourth Position

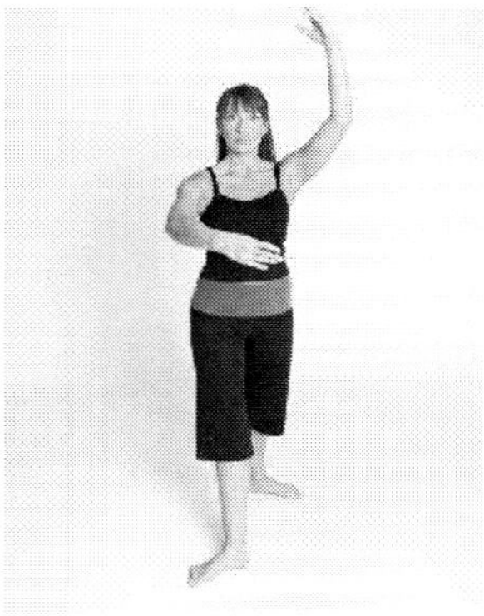

Legs - The placement of the feet is similar to the Third position but the feet are apart. The front leg moves forward about one foot distance apart. An open position like Second position.

Arms – As for Third position, the arms work in opposition to the feet. Raise the left arm up (as for Third position) and bring the right arm in front of the body, level to the navel (as for First position).

Fifth Position

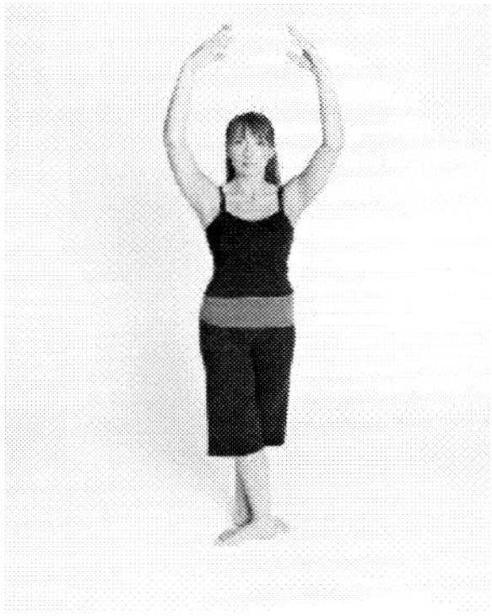

Legs – One leg is crossed directly in front of the other so that the feet are therefore running parallel with each other in a turned out position (i.e. the heel of the front foot touches and is level to the toes of the opposite foot and vice versa).

Arms – From First position, raise the arms up (not directly above the head but slightly forward) maintaining the same soft arc shape with the elbows soft and fingers long. The palms face inwards and are approximately six inches apart.

Battements Tendu

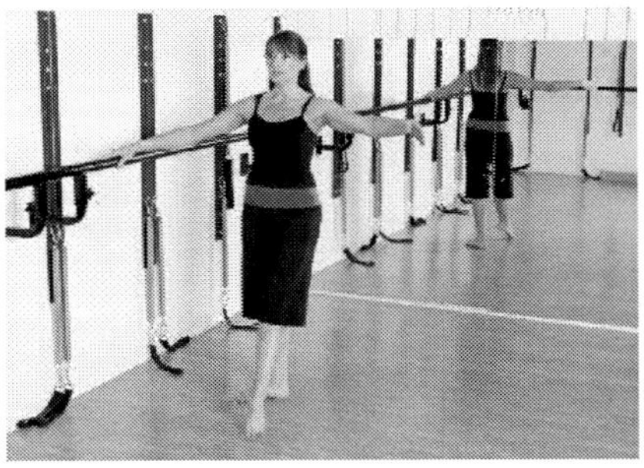

Aim

This is a preparatory exercise for battement glissé or degagé. It strengthens the feet.

Starting position

Stand upright in Fifth position. One hand is on the barre and the other hand is held out in Second position.

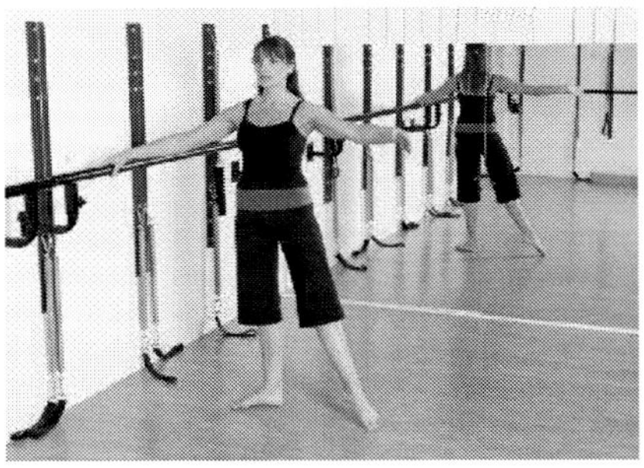

Action

Inhale – engage the core abdominals and lengthen up tall

Exhale – to point the front foot forwards directly in front of the body, maintaining the external rotation of the leg in the hip socket and a stable pelvis. The toe is pointed and remains on the floor.

Inhale – to draw the leg back to fifth position again

Exhale – point the foot out to the side this time, maintaining the external rotation of the leg with the pelvis level and stable. The arm remains in second position.

Inhale – to draw the leg back again. The working leg crosses behind the supporting leg.

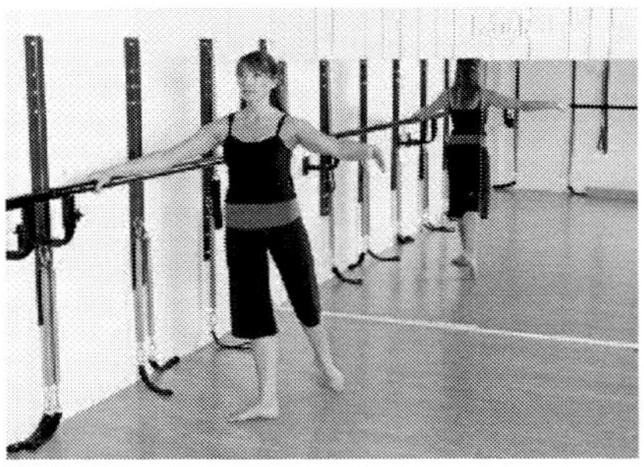

Exhale – point the foot behind and to the back, maintaining the external rotation of the leg with the pelvis level and stable. The arm remains in second position.

Inhale – to draw the leg back in again

Exhale – point the foot out to the side this time, maintaining the external rotation of the leg with the pelvis level and stable. The arm remains in second position.

Inhale – to draw the leg back in again. The working leg crosses in front of the supporting leg.

Target Muscles

Quadriceps, core abdominals, adductors, gluteals, lateral rotators

Watchpoints

- Ensure the pelvis stays level throughout so both ASIS are level
- Maintain equal length on both sides of the waist
- Ensure that the knee caps of both legs are pulled up but not locked out
- Maintain good scapula stability, with ears away from the shoulders
- Use the core abdominals well so that the spine maintains stability

Contra-indications

A turned out position may not be suitable for those with sciatica

Battements Glissé

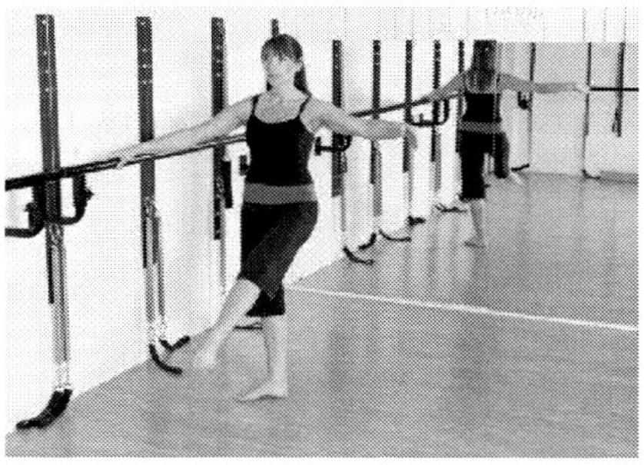

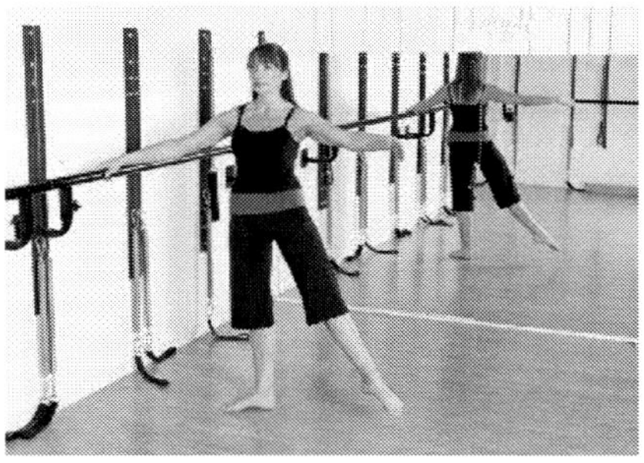

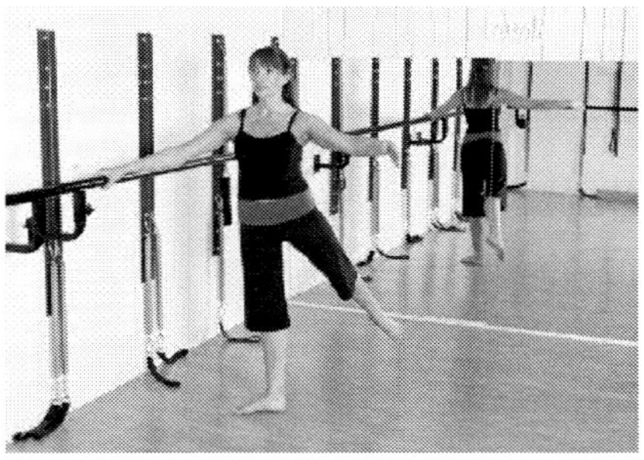

Aim

This is a progression from battements tendu and a preparatory exercise for grand battements. It strengthens the feet and legs and has a strong quality of movement and therefore a greater degree of control is required. The accent is on the returning phase of the movement, drawing the leg inwards.

Starting position

Stand upright in Fifth position. One hand is on the barre and the other hand is held out in Second position.

Action

Inhale – engage the core abdominals and lengthen up tall

Exhale – to slide the front leg forwards directly in front of the body, maintaining the external rotation of the leg in the hip socket and a stable pelvis. The foot lifts off the floor by approximately four inches.

Inhale – to glide the leg back to the floor again in a sharp, controlled manner, passing through battement tendu before the feet close together again

Exhale – slide the leg out to the side this time, maintaining the external rotation of the leg with the pelvis level and stable. The arm remains in second position.

Inhale – to glide the leg back again. The working leg crosses behind the supporting leg.

Exhale – slide the leg behind and to the back, maintaining the external rotation of the leg with the pelvis level and stable. The arm remains in second position.

Inhale – to glide the leg back in again

Exhale – slide out to the side this time, maintaining the external rotation of the leg with the pelvis level and stable. The arm remains in second position.

Inhale – to glide the leg back in again. The working leg crosses in front of the supporting leg.

Target Muscles

Quadriceps, core abdominals, adductors, gluteals, lateral rotators, hip flexors

Watchpoints

- Ensure the pelvis stays level throughout so both ASIS are level
- Maintain equal length on both sides of the waist
- Ensure that the knee caps of both legs are pulled up but not locked out
- Maintain good scapula stability, with ears away from the shoulders
- Use the core abdominals well so that the spine maintains stability
- Ensure that the leg passes through the tendu position and the accent of the movement is on the downward phase

Contra-indications

A turned out position may not be suitable for those with sciatica

Grand Battements

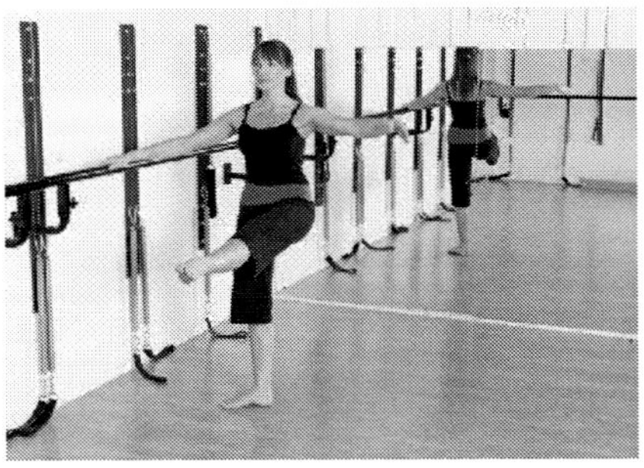

Aim

This is a strong exercise, where the leg is lifted much higher than in the battements glissé, which requires great control so that the leg is not thrown up into the air. There is great potential for pelvic movement here, so ensure that the core abdominals are engaged and the range of movement is limited to where the pelvis remains stable. The leg should appear to move with relative ease. The accent is on the downward movement of the leg.

Starting position

Stand upright in Fifth position. One hand is on the barre and the other hand is held out in Second position.

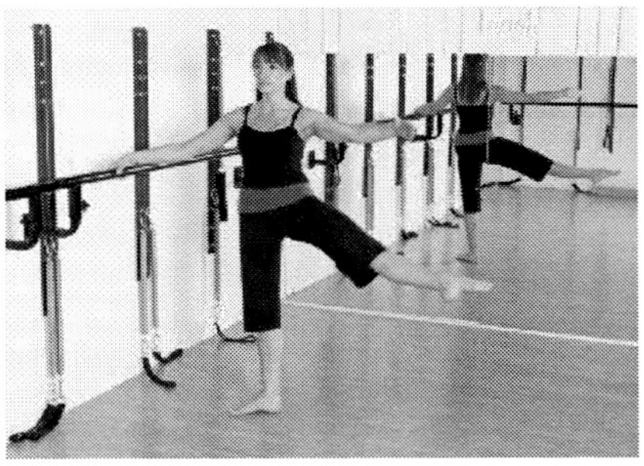

Action

Inhale – engage the core abdominals and lengthen up tall

Exhale – to quickly extend the front leg forwards directly in front of the body, maintaining the external rotation of the leg in the hip socket and a stable pelvis

Inhale – to quickly lower the leg back to the floor again in a sharp, controlled manner, passing through battement tendu before the feet close together again

Exhale – extend the leg out to the side this time, maintaining the external rotation of the leg with the pelvis level and stable. The arm remains in second position.

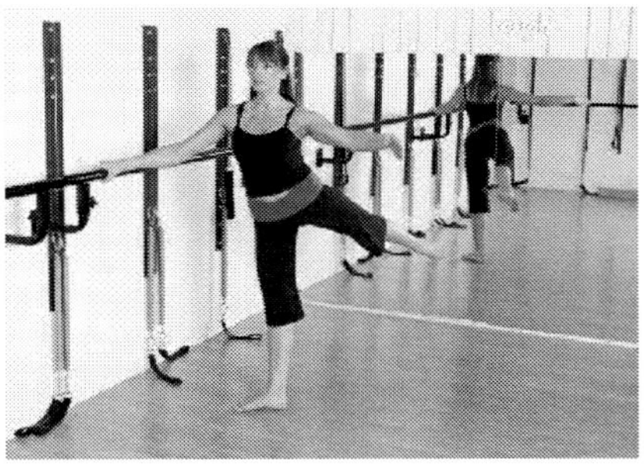

Inhale – to quickly lower the leg back to the floor again in a sharp, controlled manner, passing through battement tendu before the feet close together again. The working leg crosses behind the supporting leg.

Exhale – extend the leg behind and to the back, maintaining the external rotation of the leg with the pelvis level and stable. The arm remains in second position.

Inhale – to quickly lower the leg back to the floor again in a sharp, controlled manner, passing through battement tendu before the feet close together again

Exhale – extend the leg out to the side this time, maintaining the external rotation of the leg with the pelvis level and stable. The arm remains in second position.

Inhale – to quickly lower the leg back to the floor again in a sharp, controlled manner, passing through battement tendu before the feet close together again. The working leg crosses in front of the supporting leg.

Target Muscles

Quadriceps, core abdominals, hamstrings, adductors, gluteals, lateral rotators, hip flexors

Watchpoints

- Ensure the pelvis stays level throughout so both ASIS are level
- Maintain equal length on both sides of the waist
- Ensure that the knee caps of both legs are pulled up but not locked out
- Maintain good scapula stability, with ears away from the shoulders
- Keep the external rotation of the leg throughout, particularly as the leg extends laterally to avoid the natural tendency to turn in. If this is difficult, then limit the range of movement and height of the leg
- Use the core abdominals well so that the spine maintains stability
- Do not swing or throw the leg – the movement quality is strong, sharp and controlled yet appears to move with apparent ease
- Ensure that the leg passes through the tendu position and the accent of the movement is on the downward phase

Contra-indications

A turned out position may not be suitable for those with sciatica

Pliés in Parallel

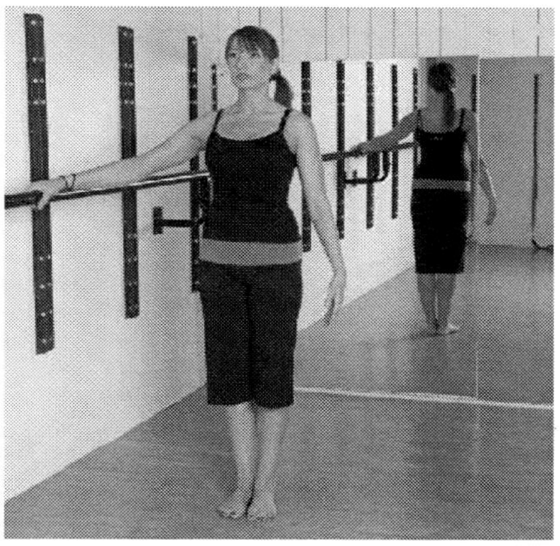

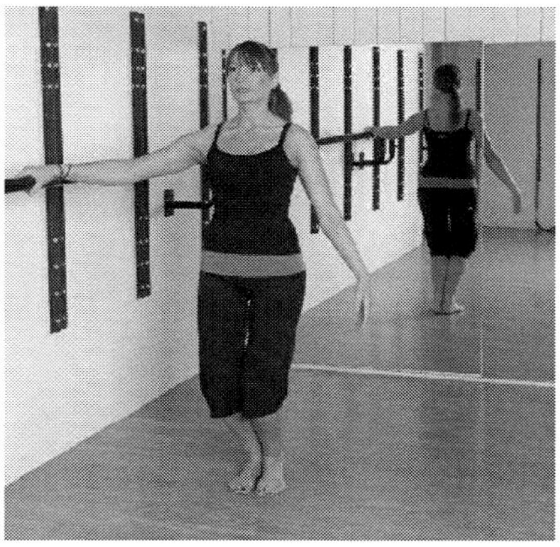

Aim

To work the quadriceps and stretch the achilles, whilst maintaining an upright posture and neutral pelvis

Starting position

Stand upright in a parallel stance with the feet and legs adducted together. The spine is in a neutral position. One hand is on the barre and the other hand is down by the side.

Action

Inhale – to prepare and lengthen the body

Exhale – engage the core abdominals and bend the knees, maintaining engagement of the adductor muscles and ensuring that the heels remain on the floor

Inhale – to extend the knees again, keeping the abdominals hollowed

Target Muscles

Quadriceps, core abdominals, soleus, adductors, gluteals

Watchpoints

- Try not to let the heels come off the floor as the knees flex
- Try not to stick out the buttocks as the knees flex to ensure a neutral spine is maintained
- Ensure an even weight distribution at the feet to avoid any rolling in or out on the ankle

Pliés in Parallel on the Toes

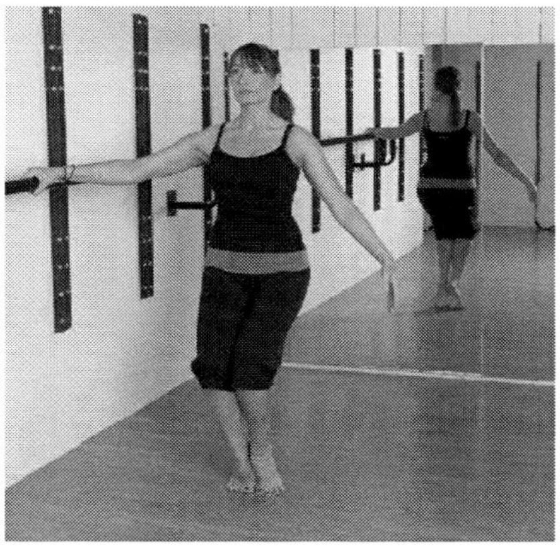

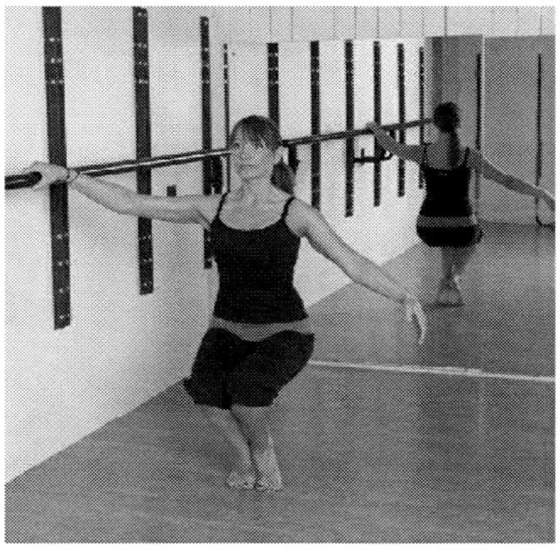

Aim

To work the quadriceps and stretch the achilles, whilst maintaining an upright posture and neutral pelvis

Starting position

Stand upright in a parallel stance with the feet and legs adducted together. The spine is in a neutral position. Relevé onto demi pointe with the heels high off the ground. One hand is on the barre and the other hand is in a low second position.

Action

Inhale – to prepare and lengthen the body

Exhale – engage the core abdominals and bend the knees, maintaining engagement of the adductor muscles and ensuring that the heels remain off the floor

Inhale – to extend the knees again, keeping the abdominals hollowed

Target Muscles

Quadriceps, core abdominals, soleus, adductors, gluteals, gastrocnemus

Watchpoints

- Try not to let the heels lower as the knees flex
- Try not to stick out the buttocks as the knees flex to ensure a neutral spine is maintained
- Ensure an even weight distribution at the feet to avoid any rolling in or out on the ankle
- Ensure that the collar bones are open, neck long and shoulders relaxed

Pliés in First position in turn out

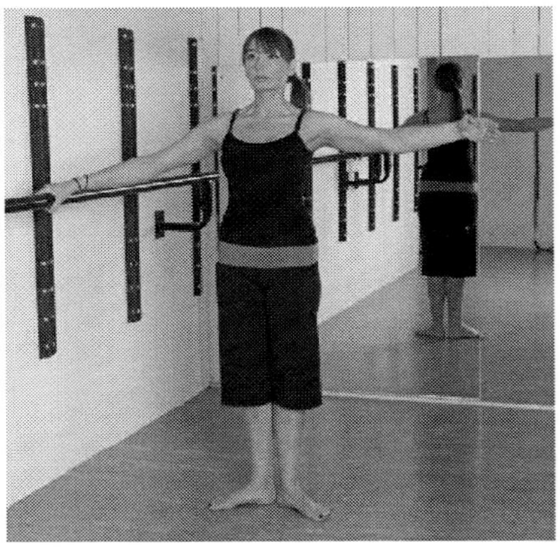

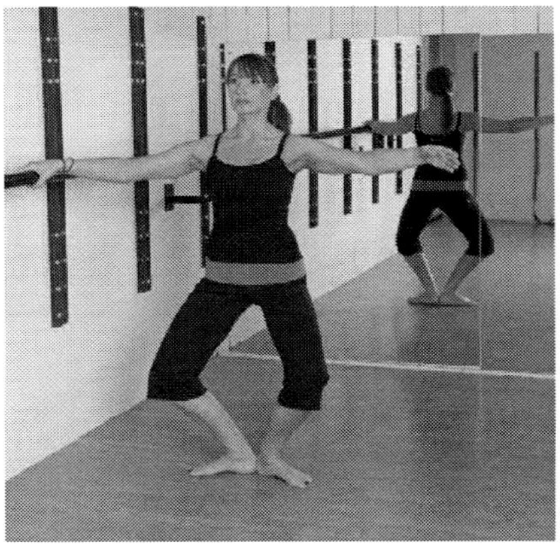

Aim

To work in external rotation. The turned out position of the leg emphasises more work from the adductors and gluteals.

Starting position

Stand upright in first position with the toes apart and the heels together. The legs are laterally rotated from the hip socket. One hand is on the barre and the other hand is in second position.

Action

Inhale – to prepare and lengthen the body

Exhale – engage the core abdominals and bend the knees, ensuring that the heels remain on the floor

Inhale – to extend the knees again

Target Muscles

Quadriceps, core abdominals, soleus, adductors, gluteals, lateral rotators

Watchpoints

- Try not to let the heels come apart or off the floor during this exercise
- Keep the knee in line with the 2nd toe to avoid the knees rolling in
- Try not to stick out the buttocks as the knees flex to ensure a neutral spine is maintained

Contra-indications

A turned out position may not be suitable for those with sciatia

Pliés in First position in turn out on the toes

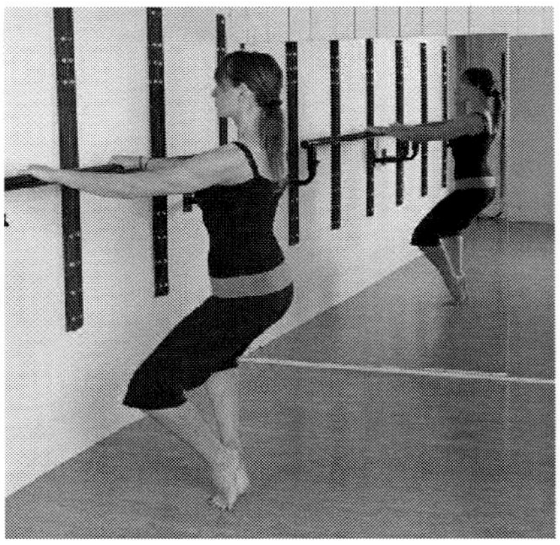

Aim

To work in external rotation again. This version is more challenging than the previous exercise, since it requires more work from the quadriceps and gastrocnemus.

Starting position

Stand upright in first position with the toes apart and the heels together. The legs are laterally rotated from the hip socket. Elevé onto the tip toes, keeping the heels together and the legs adducted. One hand is on the barre and the other hand is in first position. Alternatively, this may be done facing the barre, with both hands on the barre (as shown).

Action

Inhale – to prepare and lengthen the body

Exhale – engage the core abdominals and bend the knees, ensuring that the heels stay together

Inhale – to extend the knees again

Target Muscles

Quadriceps, core abdominals, gastrocnemius, soleus, adductors, gluteals, lateral rotators

Watchpoints

- Try not to let the heels come apart during this exercise
- Keep the knee in line with the 2nd toe to avoid the knees rolling in
- Try not to stick out the buttocks as the knees flex to ensure a neutral spine is maintained

Contra-indications

A turned out position may not be suitable for those with sciatica

Pliés in Second position in turn out

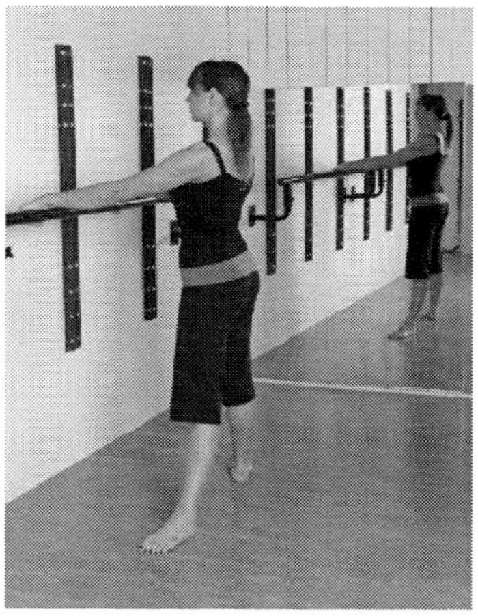

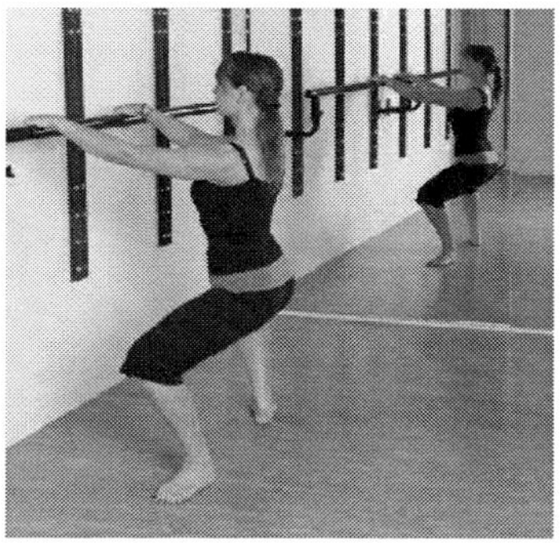

Aim

To work in external rotation. The turned out position of the leg emphasises more work from the adductors and gluteals than in first position.

Starting position

Stand upright in first position with the toes apart and the heels together. The legs are laterally rotated from the hip socket. Tendu the outside leg out to second position. One hand is on the barre and the other hand is held out in second position. Alternatively, this may be done facing the barre, with both hands on the barre (as shown).

Action

Inhale – to prepare and lengthen the body

Exhale – engage the core abdominals and bend the knees, ensuring that the heels remain on the floor

Inhale – to extend the knees again

Target Muscles

Quadriceps, core abdominals, soleus, adductors, gluteals, lateral rotators

Watchpoints

- Try not to let the heels come off the floor during this exercise
- Keep the knee in line with the 2nd toe to avoid the knees rolling in
- Try not to stick out the buttocks as the knees flex to ensure a neutral spine is maintained

Contra-indications

A turned out position may not be suitable for those with sciatica

Pliés in Second position in turn out on the toes

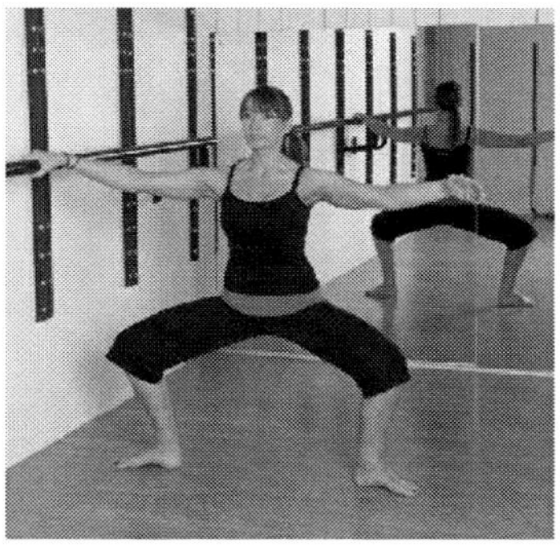

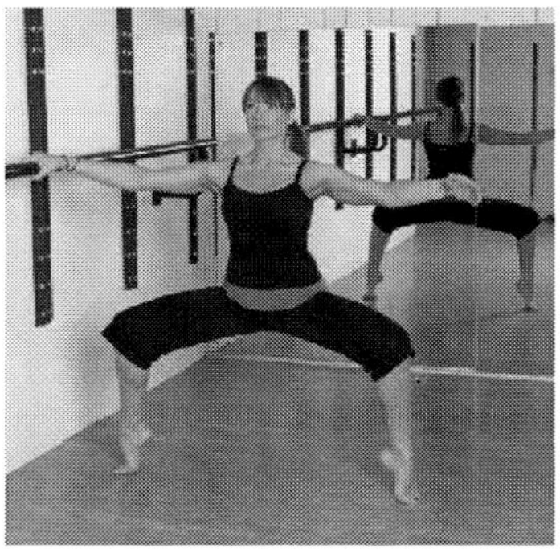

Aim

To work in external rotation. The turned out position of the leg emphasises more work from the adductors and gluteals. This version is more challenging than the previous exercise, since it requires more work from the quadriceps and gastrocnemus.

Starting position

Stand upright in first position with the toes apart and the heels together. The legs are laterally rotated from the hip socket. Tendu the outside leg out to second position. Elevé onto the tip toes. One hand is on the barre and the other hand is in second position.

Action

Inhale – to prepare and lengthen the body

Exhale – engage the core abdominals and bend the knees, ensuring that the heels remain in the same position throughout and do not drop

Inhale – to extend the knees again

Target Muscles

Quadriceps, core abdominals, gastrocnemius, soleus, adductors, gluteals, lateral rotators

Watchpoints

- Try not to let the heels drop during this exercise
- Keep the knee in line with the 2nd toe to avoid the knees rolling in
- Try not to stick out the buttocks as the knees flex to ensure a neutral spine is maintained

Contra-indications

A turned out position may not be suitable for those with sciatica

Fondue (Single leg Pliés) in First position in turn out

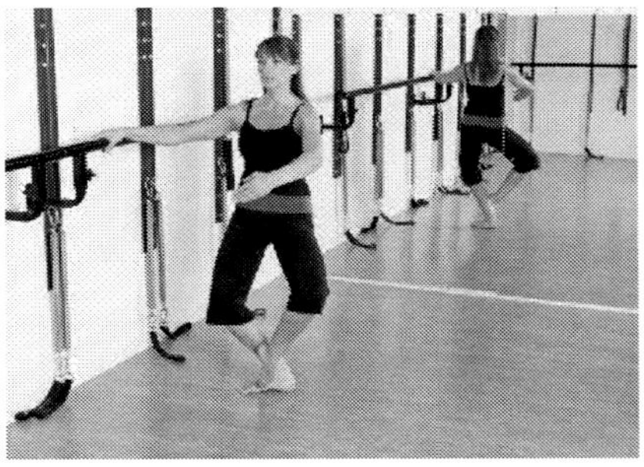

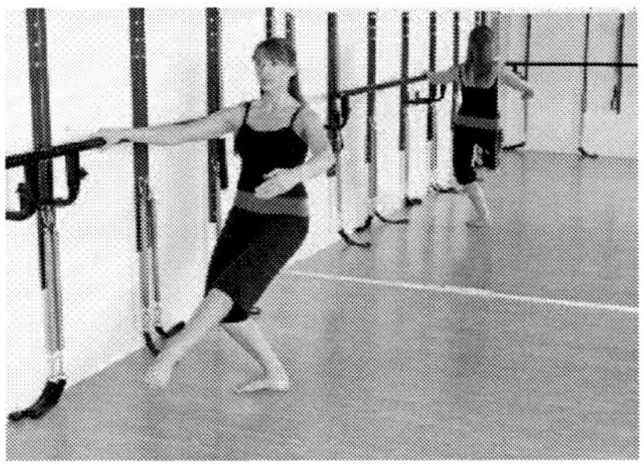

Aim

Single leg plies are much more challenging since one leg only is doing the work.

Starting position

Stand upright in first position with the toes apart and the heels together. The legs are laterally rotated from the hip socket. One hand is on the barre and the other hand is in first position. Bend both knees but allow the foot of the working leg to come off the floor as shown.

Action

Inhale – to prepare and lengthen the body

Exhale – engage the core abdominals and extend the working knee, ensuring that the heel of the supporting leg remains on the floor

Inhale – to extend the knee of the supporting leg again, whilst flexing the knee of the working leg

Target Muscles

Quadriceps, core abdominals, soleus, adductors, gluteals, lateral rotators, hip flexors

- **Watchpoints**
- Keep the knee in line with the 2nd toe to avoid the knee rolling in
- Try not to stick out the buttocks as the knee flexes to ensure a neutral spine is maintained
- Maintain a stable pelvis and the waist long and even on both sides
- Maintain the position of the leg off the floor throughout

Adaptation

This may be done in a parallel position

Contra-indications

A turned out position may not be suitable for those with sciatica

Fondue (Single leg Pliés) in First position in turn out on the toes

Aim

The workload for the quadriceps and gastrocnemus is much harder here

Starting position

Stand upright in first position with the toes apart and the heels together. The legs are laterally rotated. Relevé onto both tip toes. Degagé the outside leg and hold it a few inches from the floor to either the front or side.

Action

Inhale – to prepare and lengthen the body

Exhale – engage the core abdominals and bend both knees, ensuring that the heels remain **off** the floor

Inhale – to extend the knee again

Target Muscles

Quadriceps, gastrocnemus, soleus, adductors, gluteals, lateral rotators, hip flexors

Watchpoints

- Keep the knee in line with the 2nd toe to avoid the knee rolling in
- Try not to stick out the buttocks as the knee flexes to maintain a neutral spine
- Maintain a stable pelvis and the waist long and even on both sides
- Maintain the position of the leg off the floor throughout

Adaptation

This may be done in a parallel position

Elevé - Single elevés in Parallel

Aim

To strengthen the calves

Starting position

Stand upright in a parallel stance with the legs and feet together. Relevé (rise up onto demi ponte) onto the tip toes. One hand is on the barre and the other hand is in first position.

Action

Inhale – to prepare and lengthen the body and move the arm out to second position

Exhale – engage the core abdominals and bend one knee, whilst remaining on the tip toe of the other leg

Inhale – to extend the knee again so you are once again on both tip toes

Exhale – to repeat with the opposite leg. Alternate from one foot to the other.

Target Muscles

Quadriceps, core abdominals, soleus, gastrocnemus, adductors, gluteals,

Watchpoints

- Try to avoid hip hiking when transferring from one foot to the other. The waist should remain long and equal on both sides
- Keep the ASIS level on each side to ensure that the pelvis remains stable
- Try not to stick out the buttocks as the knees flex to maintain a neutral spine
- Ensure correct alignment of the ankle, knee and hip
- Try to lengthen the body and create a sense of opposition whilst moving to avoid shortening in the neck and shoulders. Keep the collar bones open.
- Ensure that there is no rolling inwards or outwards of the feet or ankles. Try to keep an even weight distribution across the entire foot
- Ensure that a full range of motion is achieved so the feet are worked fully
- Ensure that both legs are working equally
- Maintain a sense of inner thigh and sit bone connection

Variation One - Single elevés in First Position in turn out

Variation Two - Single elevés in Second Position in turn out

Contraindications – A turned out position may not be suitable for sciatica

Double Elevés

Aim

To strengthen the calves

Starting position

Stand upright in a parallel stance with the legs and feet together. One hand is on the barre and the other hand is in first position.

Action

Inhale – to prepare and lengthen the body and move the arm out to second position

Exhale – engage the core abdominals and relevé onto both tip toes

Inhale – to lower back down onto the heels again

Target Muscles

Quadriceps, core abdominals, soleus, gastrocnemus, adductors, gluteals,

Watchpoints

- Keep the ASIS level on each side to ensure that the pelvis remains stable
- Try not to stick out the buttocks and ensure a neutral spine is maintained
- Ensure correct alignment of the ankle, knee and hip
- Try to lengthen the body and create a sense of opposition whilst moving to avoid shortening in the neck and shoulders. Keep the collar bones open.
- Ensure that there is no rolling inwards or outwards of the feet or ankles.
- Ensure that a full range of motion is achieved so the feet are worked fully
- Maintain a sense of inner thigh and sit bone connection

Variation One - Double elevés in First Position in turn out

Variation Two - Double elevés in Second Position in turn out

Contraindications – A turned out position may not be suitable for sciatica

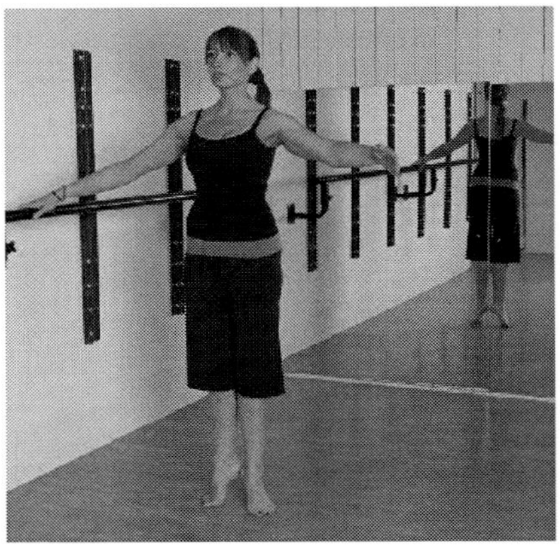

Variation One

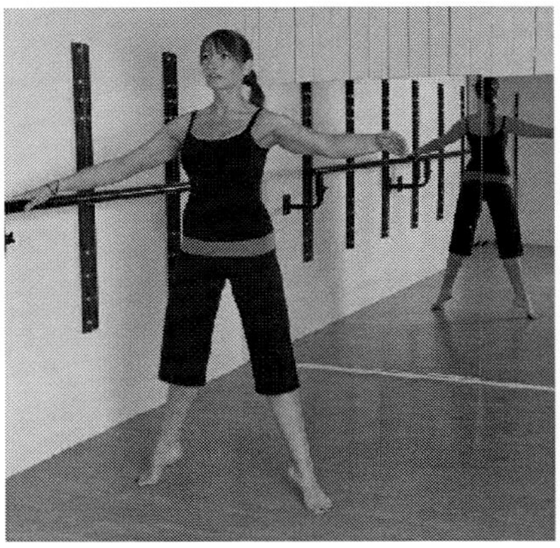

Variation Two

Single Relevés in Parallel

Aim

To strengthen the calves and quadriceps

Starting position

Stand upright in a parallel stance with the legs and feet together. Elevé onto the tip toes. Bend both knees into a demi plie. One hand is on the barre and the other hand is in first position.

Action

Inhale – to prepare and lengthen the body and move the arm out to second position

Exhale – engage the core abdominals and lower one heel to the floor, whilst remaining on the tip toe of the other foot

Inhale – to raise the heel again so you are once again on both tip toes

Exhale – to repeat with the opposite leg. Alternate from one heel to the other.

Target Muscles

Quadriceps, core abdominals, soleus, adductors, gluteals, gastrocnemus

Watchpoints

- Try to avoid hip hiking when transferring from one foot to the other. The waist should remain long and equal on both sides
- The buttocks and the head should remain at the same height throughout
- Keep the ASIS level on each side to ensure that the pelvis remains stable
- Try to lengthen the body and create a sense of opposition whilst moving to avoid shortening in the neck and shoulders. Keep the collar bones open.
- Ensure that there is no rolling inwards or outwards of the feet or ankles. Try to keep an even weight distribution across the entire foot
- Ensure that a full range of motion is achieved so the feet are worked fully
- Ensure that both legs are working equally

Variation One - Single Relevés in First Position in turn out in Plie

Variation Two - Single Relevés in Second Position in turn out in Plie

Contraindications – A turned out position may not be suitable for sciatica

Double Relevés in Parallel

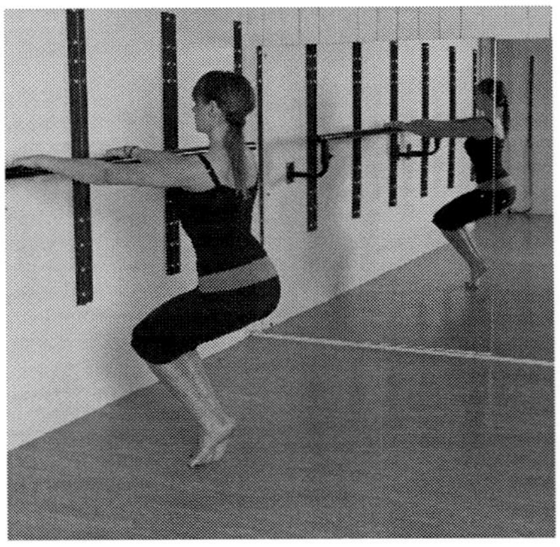

Aim

To strengthen the calves and quadriceps

Starting position

Stand upright in a parallel stance with the legs and feet together. Bend both knees into a demi plie. One hand is on the barre and the other hand is in first position. Alternatively, this may be done facing the barre, with both hands on the barre (as shown).

Action

Inhale – to prepare and lengthen the body and move the arm out to second position

Exhale – engage the core abdominals and relevé onto both tip toes

Inhale – to lower back down onto the heels again

Target Muscles

Quadriceps, core abdominals, soleus, gastrocnemus, adductors, gluteals,

Watchpoints

- The waist should remain long and equal on both sides
- The buttocks and the head should remain at the same height throughout
- Keep the ASIS level on each side to ensure that the pelvis remains stable
- Try to lengthen the body and create a sense of opposition whilst moving to avoid shortening in the neck and shoulders. Keep the collar bones open.
- Ensure that there is no rolling inwards or outwards of the feet or ankles.
- Ensure that a full range of motion is achieved so the feet are worked fully

Variation One - Double Relevés in First Position in turn out in Plie

Variation Two - Double Relevés in Second Position in turn out in Plie

Contraindications – A turned out position may not be suitable for sciatica

Pliés with inner thigh squeeze on the toes

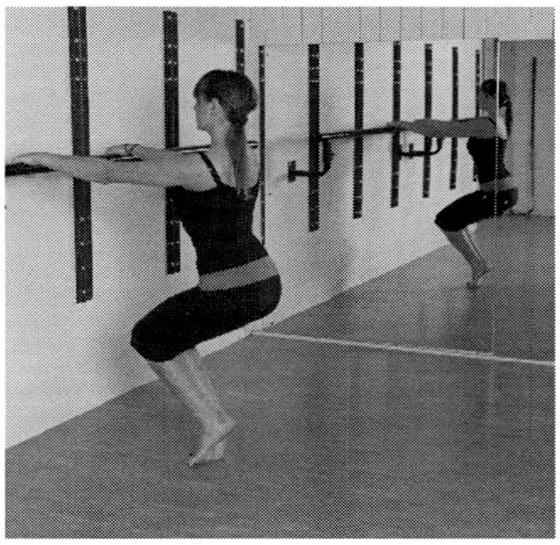

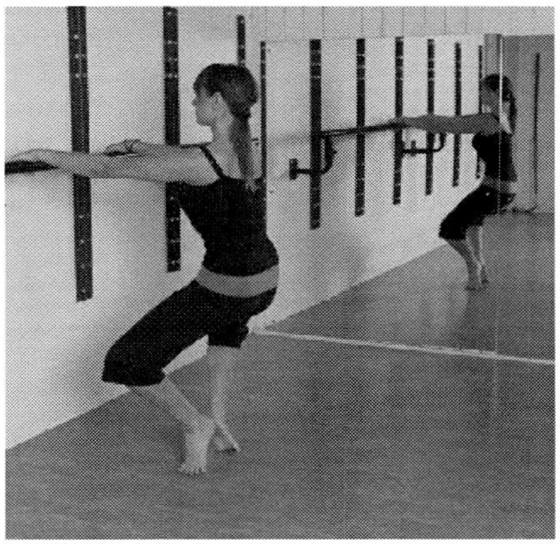

Aim

To work the adductors in conjunction with the quadriceps

Starting position

Stand upright in a parallel stance with the legs and feet together. Elevé onto the tip toes, keeping the heels together and the legs adducted. Bend the knees into a demi plié and hold this position throughout the exercise. One hand is on the barre and the other hand is in second position. Alternatively, this exercise may be done facing the barre with both hands on.

Action

Inhale – to prepare and lengthen the body

Exhale – engage the core abdominals and open out the knees as wide as a stable pelvis allows, ensuring that the heels stay together

Inhale – to close the knees again

Target Muscles

Quadriceps, core abdominals, gastrocnemius, soleus, adductors, gluteals, lateral rotators

Watchpoints

- Try not to let the heels come apart during this exercise and keep them at the same height throughout
- Keep the collar bones wide, the neck long and the shoulders relaxed
- Try to ensure a neutral spine is maintained as the legs open and close
- Ensure that there is no rolling in or out over the ankles as the legs open and close
- Keep the waist long and even on both sides

Contra-indications

A turned out position may not be suitable for those with sciatica

Pliés with pelvic tilts on the toes in Parallel

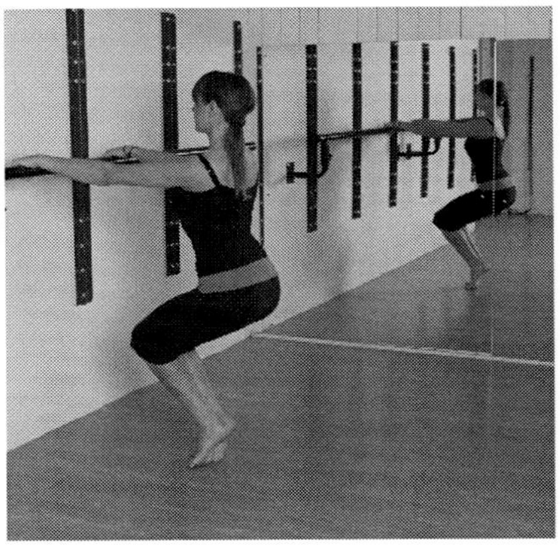

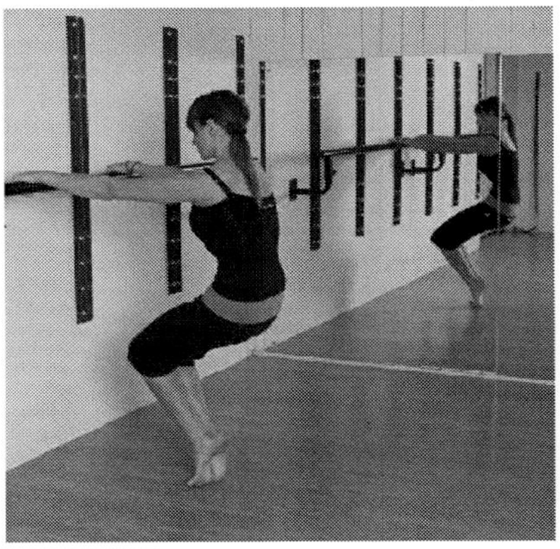

Aim

To work the gluteals in conjunction with the quadriceps

Starting position

Stand upright in a parallel stance with the legs and feet together. Elevé onto the tip toes, keeping the heels together and the legs adducted. Bend the knees into a demi plié and hold this position throughout the exercise. One hand is on the barre and the other hand is in second position. The pelvis is in a neutral position. Alternatively, this exercise may be done facing the barre with both hands on.

Action

Inhale – to prepare and lengthen the body

Exhale – engage the core abdominals and tilt the pelvis north, tucking the coccyx under, using the glutes

Inhale – to return the pelvis to a neutral position

Target Muscles

Quadriceps, core abdominals, gastrocnemius, soleus, adductors, gluteals, lateral rotators

Watchpoints

- Try not to let the heels come apart during this exercise and keep them at the same height throughout
- Keep the collar bones wide, the neck long and the shoulders relaxed
- Keep the waist long and even on both sides

Variation One – This exercise may be done in First position in turn out

Variation Two – This exercise may be done in Second position in turn out

Contra-indications

A turned out position may not be suitable for those with sciatica

Developpés

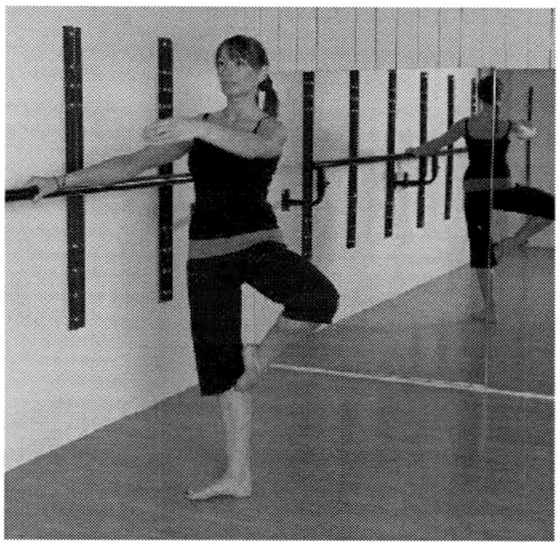

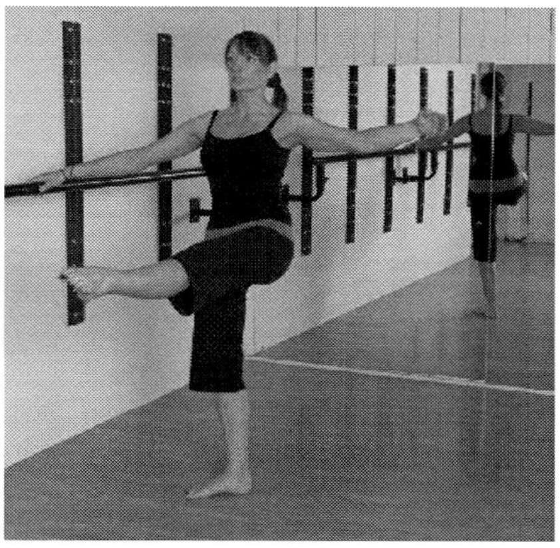

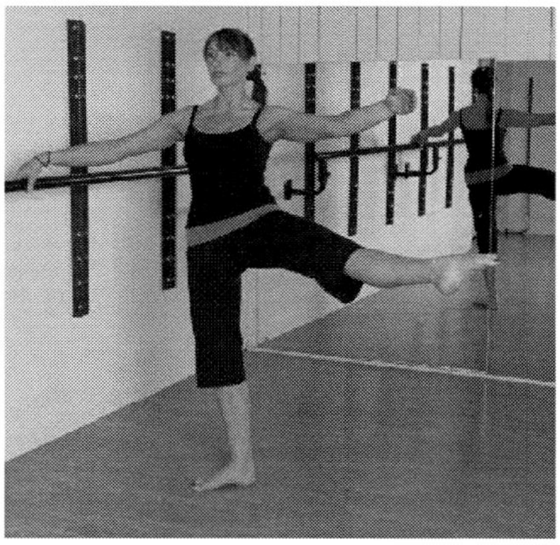

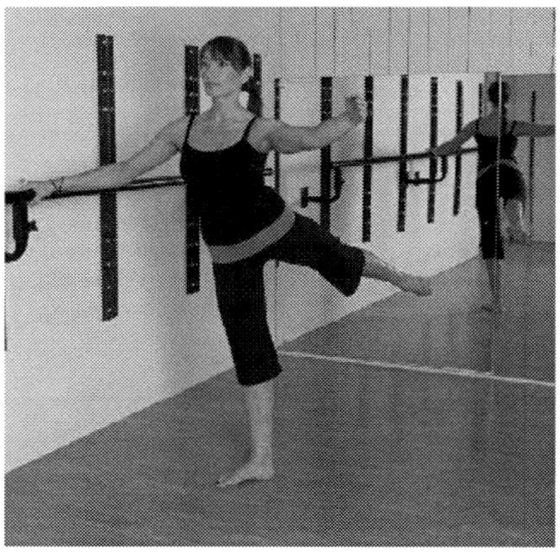

Aim

This is a complex exercise involving choreography and co-ordination. There is greater potential for pelvic movement here, so ensure that the core abdominals are engaged and the range of movement is limited to where the pelvis remains stable

Starting position

Stand upright in First position with the toes apart and the heels together. One hand is on the barre and the other hand is in bras bas.

Action

Inhale – engage the core abdominals and retiré with the outside leg so that the foot touches the opposite supporting leg at the knee. Simultaneously bring the arm up to first position.

Exhale – to extend the leg in front of the body, maintaining the external rotation of the leg in the hip socket. Simultaneously bring the arm out to second position.

Inhale – bend the knee back in so that the foot touches the inside of the knee on the supporting leg

Exhale – extend the leg out to the side this time, maintaining the external rotation of the leg with the pelvis level and stable. The arm remains in second position.

Inhale – bend the knee back in so that the foot touches the inside of the knee on the supporting leg

Exhale – extend the leg behind and to the back, maintaining the external rotation of the leg with the pelvis level and stable. Bring the arm up to fifth position (optional).

Inhale – bend the knee back in so that the foot touches the inside of the knee on the supporting leg

Exhale – to place the foot back on the floor again in first position.

Target Muscles

Quadriceps, core abdominals, hamstrings, adductors, gluteals, lateral rotators

Watchpoints

- Ensure the pelvis stays as level as possible throughout and try to maintain equal length on both sides of the waist
- Ensure that the knee caps of both legs are pulled up but not locked out
- Maintain good scapula stability, with ears away from the shoulders
- Keep the external rotation of the leg throughout, particularly as the leg extends laterally to avoid the natural tendency to turn in. If this is difficult, then limit the range of movement and height of the leg

Contra-indications

A turned out position may not be suitable for those with sciatica

Attitude

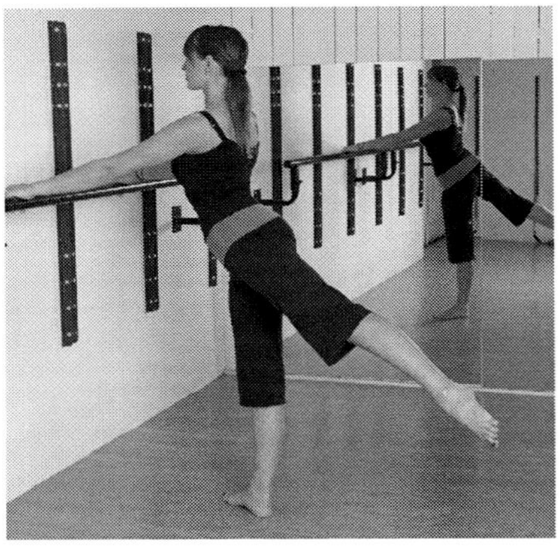

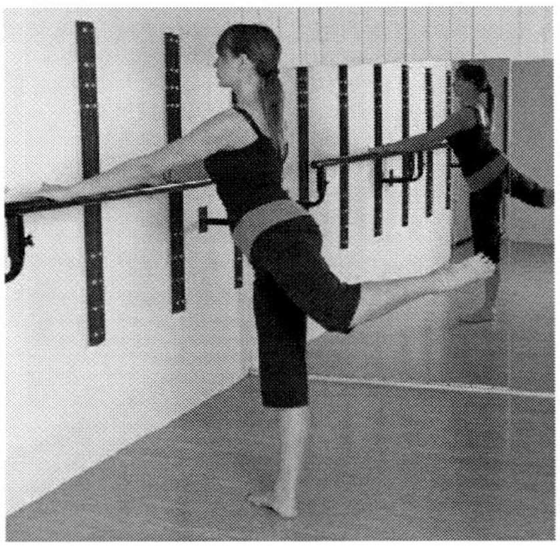

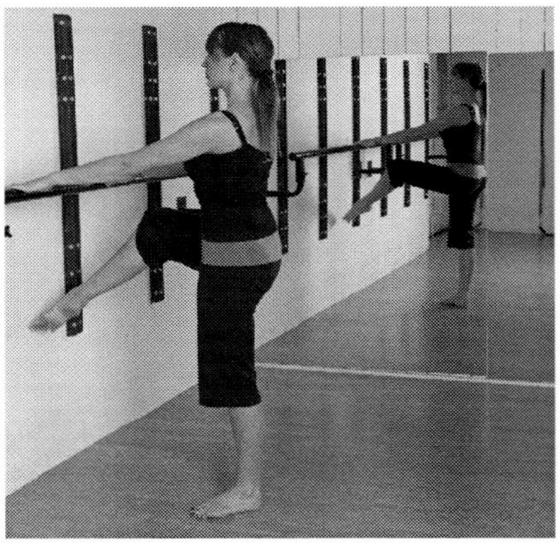

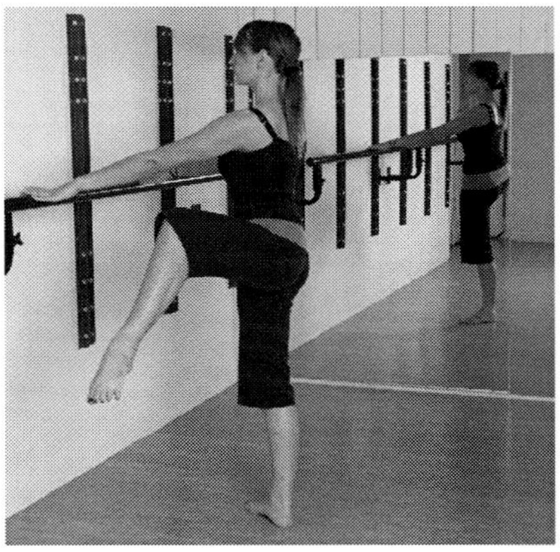

Aim

This exercise strengthens the gluteal muscles and the external rotators of the leg so requires good turnout

Starting position

Stand upright in Fifth position (left foot crossed in front), facing the barre with both hands on the barre

Action

Inhale – engage the core abdominals and lengthen up tall and raise the right arm up above the head into a fifth position and degage the right leg backwards (both hands may also remain on the barre initially)

Exhale – to bend the knee and raise the leg up. The leg is bent at 90 degrees and turned out so that the knee is higher than the foot. The body remains as stable as possible.

Inhale – to prepare

Exhale – to isometrically contract the gluteals, performing small lifting movements of no more than an inch in a pulsing like action

Inhale – to lower the leg back to the floor again when completed. Repeat with the opposite leg

Target Muscles

Core abdominals, hamstrings, gluteals, lateral rotators

Watchpoints

- Maintain good scapula stability, with ears away from the shoulders
- Keep the external rotation of the leg throughout. If this is difficult, then limit the range of movement and height of the leg. Keep the 90 degree angle of the leg and maintain the knee above the foot throughout
- Use the core abdominals well so that the spine maintains stability
- Keep the hips, shoulders and pelvis as stable as possible

Variation One

Attitudes may also be performed with the leg to the front

Variation Two

Attitudes may also be performed with the leg out to the side

Contra-indications

A turned out position may not be suitable for those with sciatica

Hamstring Curls

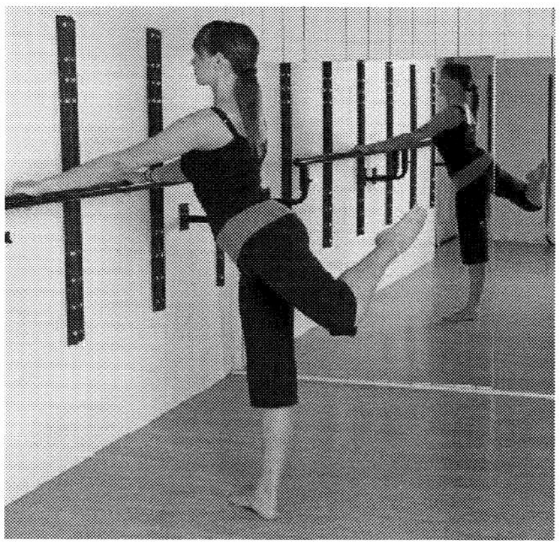

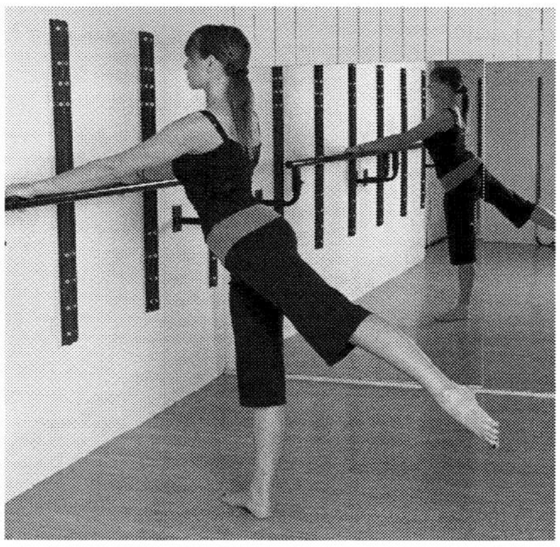

Aim

This exercise strengthens the hamstrings

Starting position

Stand upright in Fifth position (left foot crossed in front), facing the barre with both hands on the barre

Action

Exhale – engage the core abdominals and lengthen up tall and tendu the right leg backwards to come to the attitude position

Inhale – to extend the knee, maintaining the position of the knee in space.

Exhale – to flex the knee, bringing the heel towards the buttocks, whilst maintaining the position of the knee in space

Exhale – to extend the leg again. Repeat with the opposite leg

Target Muscles

Core abdominals, hamstrings, gluteals, lateral rotators

Watchpoints

- Maintain good scapula stability, with ears away from the shoulders
- Keep the external rotation of the leg throughout. If this is difficult, then limit the range of movement and height of the leg
- Use the core abdominals well so that the spine maintains stability
- Keep the hips, shoulders and pelvis as square and stable as possible
- The knee must be kept stable in the same position in space throughout

Variation One (Progression)

This exercise may be performed in a horizontal position with the torso level to the floor (as for Superman position). The legs will be in a parallel position here. The position is more challenging to maintain since the pelvic and scapula stability are harder to maintain.

Contra-indications

A turned out position may not be suitable for those with sciatica

Superman

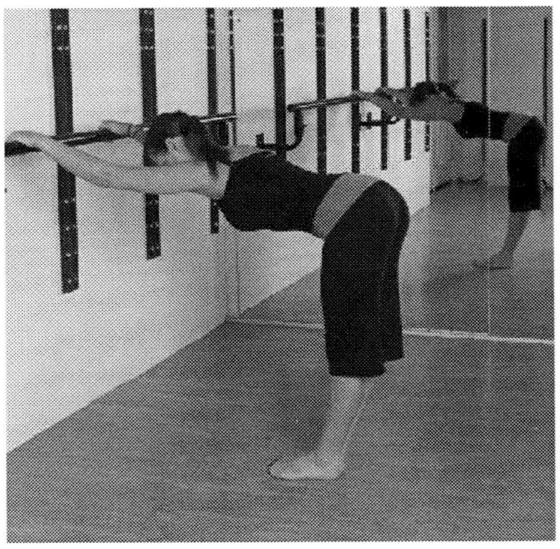

Aim

This exercise strengthens the hamstrings and gluteal muscles whilst challenging core and scapula stability

Starting position

Stand upright facing the barre with both hands on the barre, arms length away. Hinge forwards from the hips to bring the torso into a horizontal position so that the hands, shoulders and hips are all in alignment. The feet are in a parallel position

Action

Exhale – engage the core abdominals and tendu the right leg backwards and lift it up as high as a stable pelvis allows. Both ASIS should remain level. Ideally the foot should aim to be around hip height

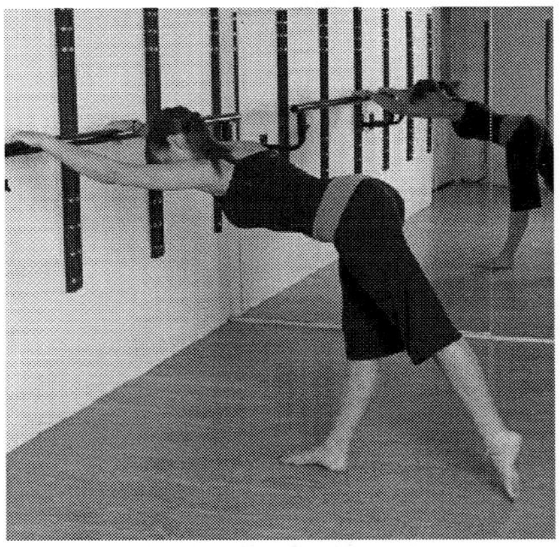

Inhale – to prepare

Exhale – to isometrically contract the gluteals and raise the leg no more than one inch in a small pulsing like motion. The leg remains in a parallel position throughout. Repeat with the opposite leg.

Target Muscles

Core abdominals, hamstrings, gluteals

Watchpoints

- Maintain good scapula stability, with ears away from the shoulders
- Use the core abdominals well so that the spine maintains length and stability
- Ensure good use of obliques to prevent the ribs from flaring
- Keep the hips, shoulders and pelvis as square and stable as possible with both ASIS's level throughout
- Ensure the supporting knee is not locked out

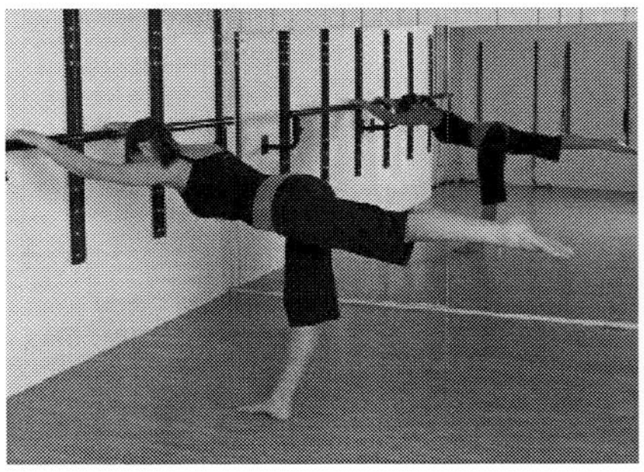

Variation One (Progression)

Abduction. Maintain the leg at hip height whilst the leg abducts a couple of inches out to the side. Adduction. Maintain the leg at hip height whilst the leg adducts in towards the midline a few inches.

Leg Abduction Variations

Side Leg Raise

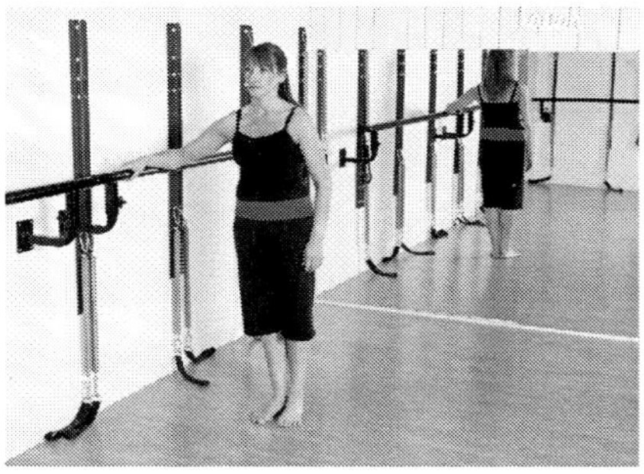

Aim

This exercise works the abductors

Starting position

Stand upright in a parallel position sideways onto the barre. One hand is on the barre and the other hand is in Second Position. Slightly lean the torso towards the barre and maintain a stable position here.

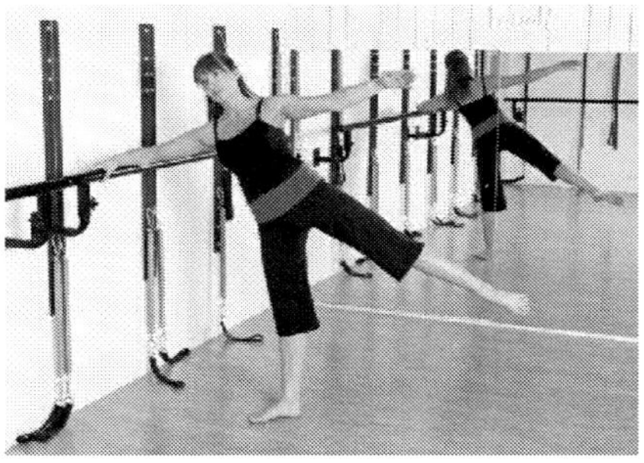

Action

Exhale – engage the core abdominals and raise the working leg out to the side and off the floor, maintaining the parallel position. Slightly lean the torso towards the barre and maintain a stable position here.

Inhale – lower the leg back towards the floor without the foot touching the floor and repeat again

Target Muscles

Glute medius and minimus, core abdominals

Watchpoints

- Ensure the pelvis stays stable throughout and keep the torso still
- Maintain equal length on both sides of the waist
- Ensure that the knee caps of both legs are pulled up but not locked out
- Maintain good scapula stability, with ears away from the shoulders

Leg Press

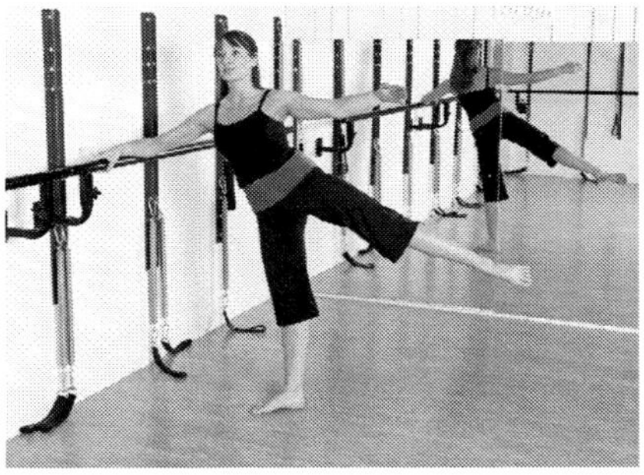

Aim

This exercise targets all of the gluteal muscles together

Starting position

Stand upright in a parallel position sideways onto the barre. One hand is on the barre and the other hand is in Second Position. Raise the working leg out to the side and off the floor, maintaining the parallel position. The elbow may rest on the barre and the torso may be inclined towards the barre.

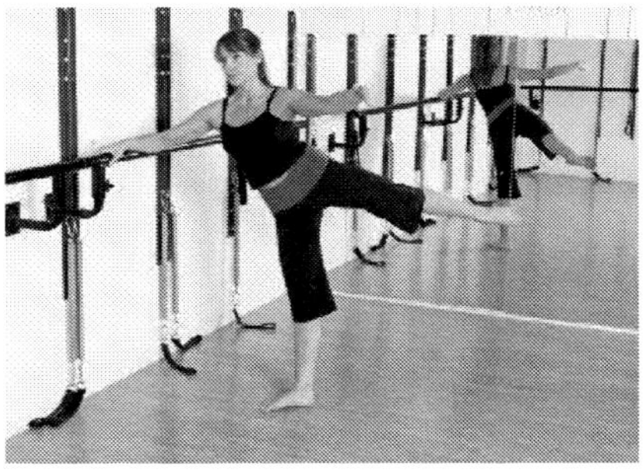

Action

Exhale – engage the core abdominals and press the working leg back behind the body a few inches, whilst keeping the leg at a constant level

Inhale – to bring it forwards again.

Target Muscles

Glute medius, minmus and maximus, core abdominals

Watchpoints

- Ensure the pelvis stays stable throughout
- Ensure that the leg remains at a constant height throughout

Leg Circles

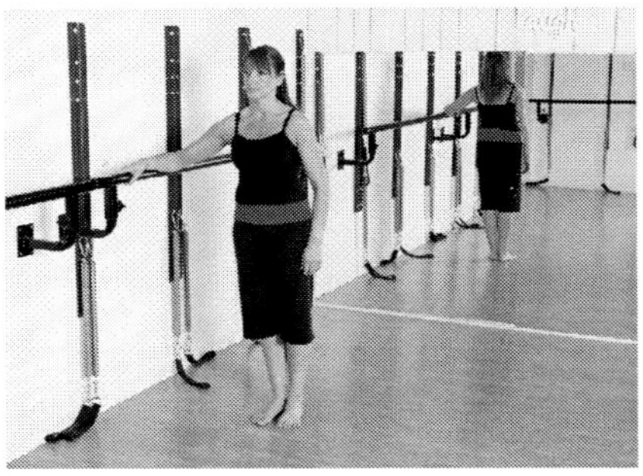

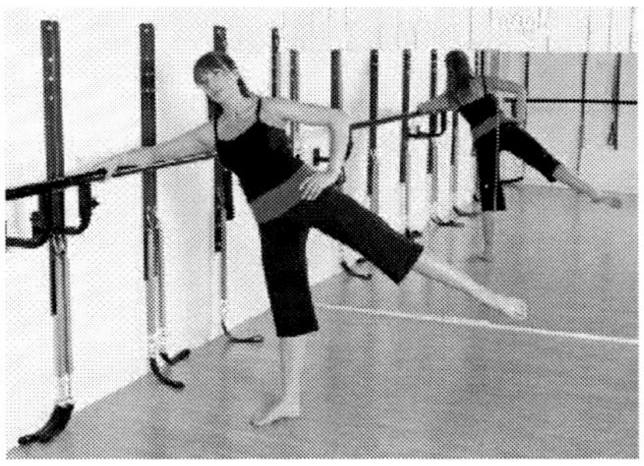

Aim

This exercise targets all of the gluteal muscles together

Starting position

Stand upright in a parallel position sideways onto the barre. One hand is on the barre and the other hand is on the hip. Side bend towards the barre, keeping the torso square. Raise the working leg out to the side and off the floor, as high as possible, maintaining the parallel position

Action

Exhale – engage the core abdominals and raise the working leg up a few inches, then press it back a few inches, lower it a few inches and finally bring it forwards and back to the start position. A small circular action is made

Inhale – to prepare and then repeat again. Then reverse the circles.

Target Muscles

Glute medius, minmus and maximus, core abdominals

Watchpoints

- Ensure the pelvis stays stable throughout
- Ensure that the torso and spine do not move as the leg moves. Use the core abdominals to aid in stability

Side Kick Karate

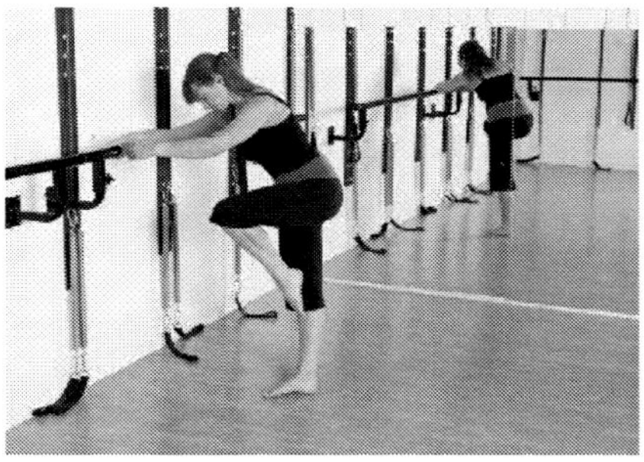

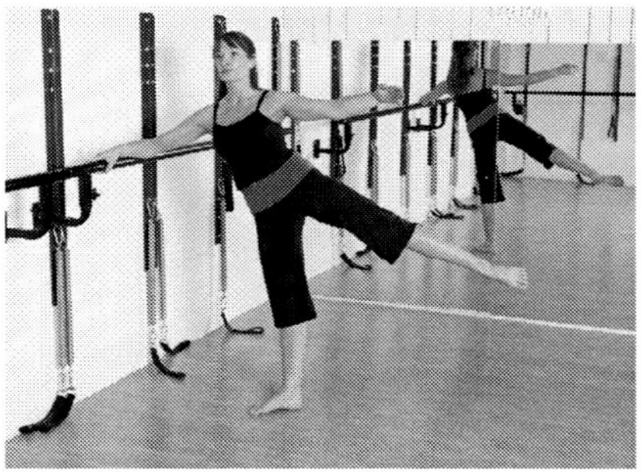

Aim

This exercise works the abductors and hamstrings

Starting position

Stand upright in a parallel position sideways onto the barre. One hand is on the barre and the other hand is in Second Position. Raise the outside arm up in the air and side bend towards the barre, keeping the torso square. Raise the working leg out to the side and off the floor, as high as possible, maintaining the parallel position

Action

Exhale – engage the core abdominals and bend the knee in towards the chest, and turn towards the barre. Keep the leg at the same height and the torso stable.

Inhale – to extend the leg back out again, pushing out through the heel and turn away from the barre again.

Target Muscles

Glute medius, minmus and maximus, core abdominals, hip flexors, hamstrings

Watchpoints

- Ensure the pelvis stays stable throughout
- Ensure that the spine stays in neutral as the leg moves. Use the core abdominals to aid in stability

Quadricep Lifts

Aim

This exercise strengthens the quadriceps and hip flexors. There is great potential for pelvic movement here, so ensure that the core abdominals are engaged and the range of movement is limited to where the pelvis remains stable.

Starting position

Sit upright on the floor with the spine resting against the wall. Place both hands on the barre and lenghten the spine as much as possible. The back may rest on the wall or may be not touch the wall as appropriate. This exercise can be performed with the spine in neutral or with slight lumbar flexion. Both legs are extended straight along the floor in parallel and adducted.

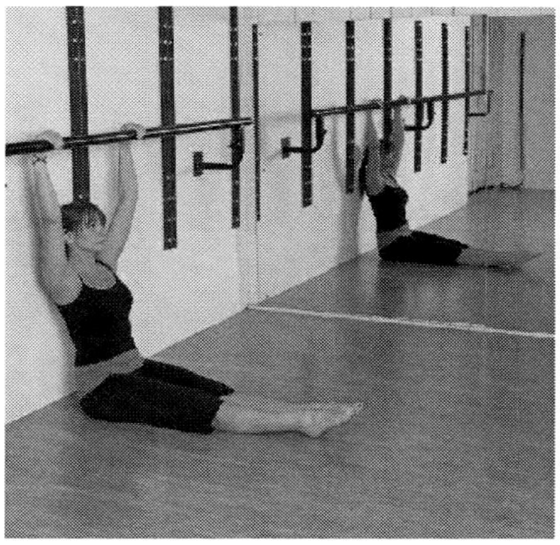

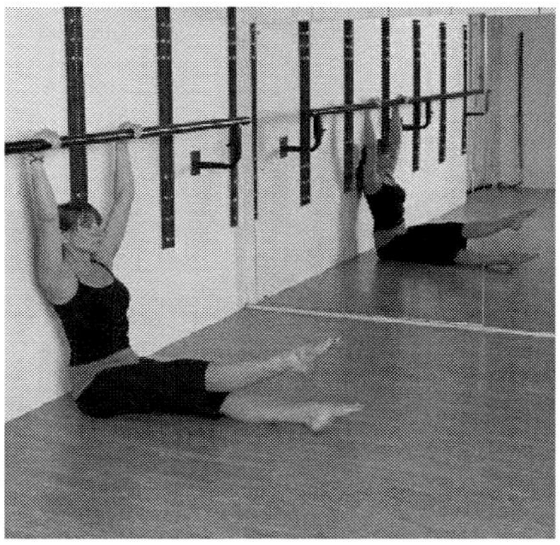

Action

Inhale – engage the core abdominals and lengthen up tall

Exhale – to raise one leg up in the air towards the barre, maintaining a stable pelvis

Inhale – to gently lower the leg back to the floor again in a controlled manner and repeat with the other leg.

Target Muscles

Quadriceps, core abdominals, hamstrings, hip flexors

Watchpoints

- Ensure the pelvis stays level throughout
- Maintain equal length on both sides of the waist
- Ensure that the knee caps of both legs are pulled up but not locked out
- Maintain good scapula stability, with ears away from the shoulders
- Ensure the lumbar spine does not get pulled into extension by the weight of the leg
- Use the core abdominals well so that the spine maintains stability
- Do not throw the leg – the movement is controlled

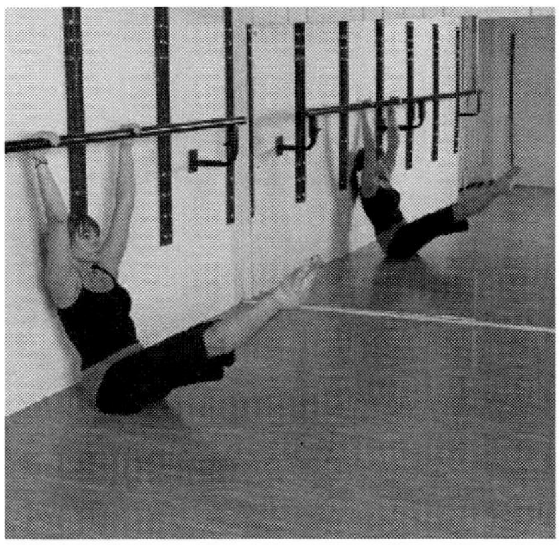

Variation Two

Variation One

This exercise may be performed with the leg in external rotation

Variation Two

This exercise may be performed lifting both legs. This is an advanced exercise, which can potentially pull on the lumbar spine. Ensure the lumbar spine does not get pulled into extension when moving the legs

Contra-indications

A turned out position may not be suitable for those with sciatica (variation one)

Press Ups

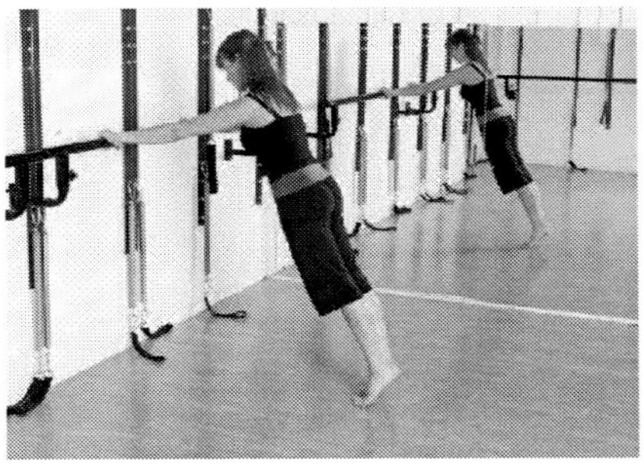

Aim

This exercise strengthens the upper body, whilst challenging core stability

Starting position

Stand upright facing the barre with the feet in a parallel position and both hands on the barre, arms length away. Move the feet back a good distance behind the shoulders (as far away as good technique allows you to perform the exercise well). The further away the feet are from the wall, the more challenging the exercise. The heels will leave the floor if the feet are far away from the wall.

Action

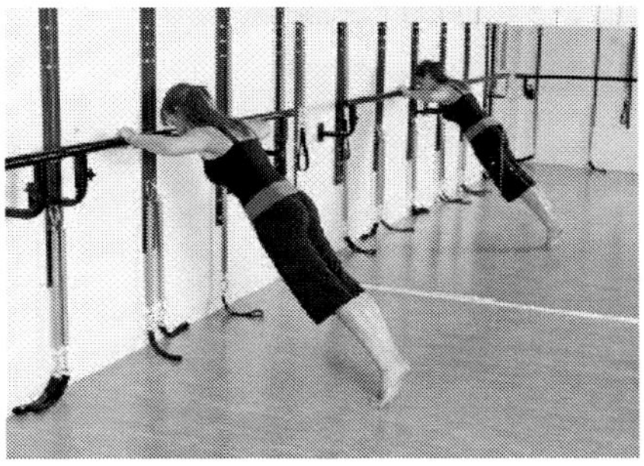

Inhale – to bend the elbows and bring the chest towards the barre, whilst maintaining spinal stability. The deeper the bend, the more challenging the exercise

Exhale – to straighten the elbows, pushing the body away from the barre

Target Muscles

Core abdominals, anterior deltoid, pectorals, triceps

Watchpoints

- Maintain good scapula stability, with ears away from the shoulders
- Keep the hips, shoulders and pelvis as square and stable as possible
- Ensure good use of core abdominals to prevent the spine from arching or losing the neutral alignment
- Ensure the buttocks do not stick out as the elbows bend
- Ensure that the movement does not come from any hinge at the waist as the elbows bend

Variation One

This exercise may be performed with one arm (single arm press ups)

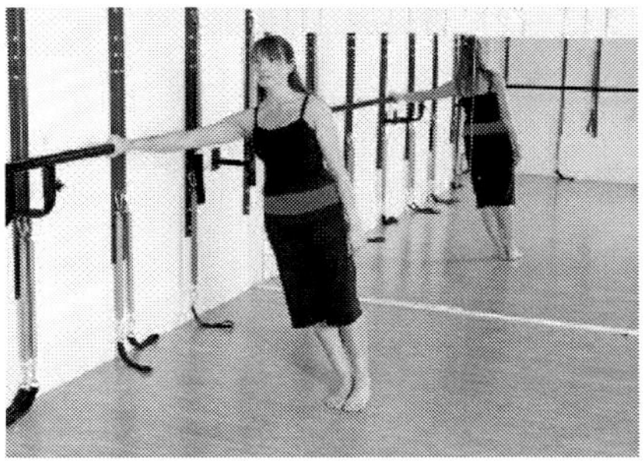

Variation One

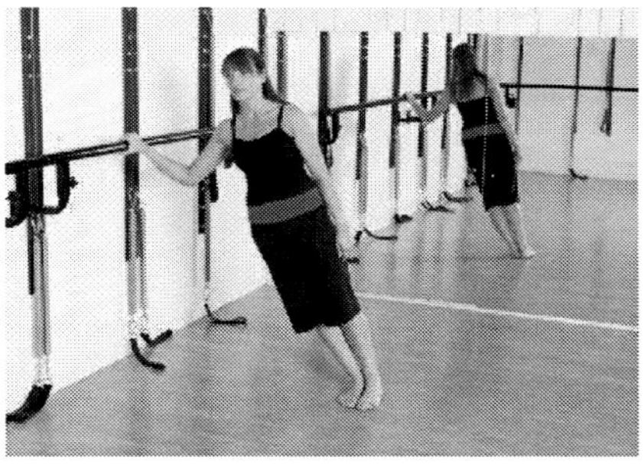

Variation One

Pull Ups

Aim

This exercise strengthens the upper body, whilst challenging core and scapula stability. It is a much more challenging exercise than the previous Press Ups version.

This exercise requires a very strong barre with secure fittings and may not be suitable to perform in a group situation due to the amount of weight exerted on the barre. A structural survey is strongly advised for this particular exercise.

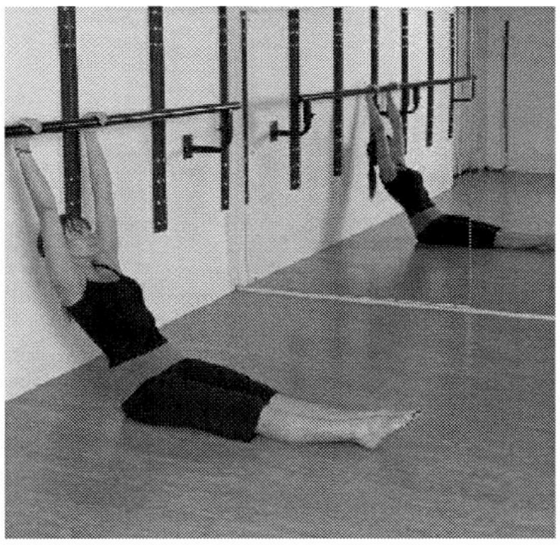

Starting position

Sit upright underneath the barre with the feet and legs together in a parallel position and place both hands on the barre, simultaneously lifting up the buttocks. The body should form a diagonal straight line from the toes to the ears. Keep the adductors and buttocks tight throughout.

Action

Exhale – to bend the elbows and pull the chest up towards the barre, whilst maintaining spinal and scapula stability. The deeper the bend, the more challenging the exercise

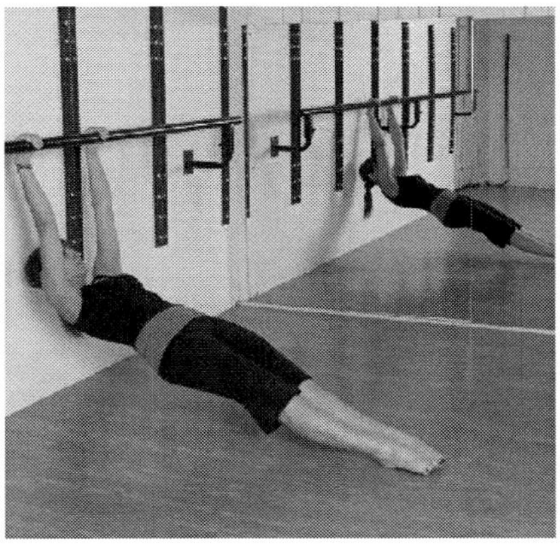

Exhale – to straighten the elbows and return to the start position, maintaining spinal stability

Target Muscles

Core abdominals, anterior deltoid, pectorals, biceps, latissimus dorsi, gluteals

Watchpoints

- Maintain good scapula stability, with ears away from the shoulders
- Keep the hips, shoulders and pelvis as square and stable as possible
- Ensure good use of core abdominals to prevent the spine from arching or losing the neutral alignment
- Ensure the gluteals are engaged so that the buttocks do not sag
- Try not to hang off the bar in between repetitions: maintain good spinal stability throughout

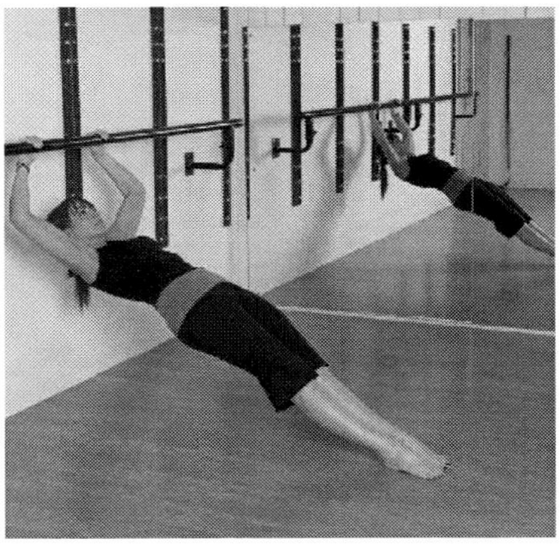

V Stretch

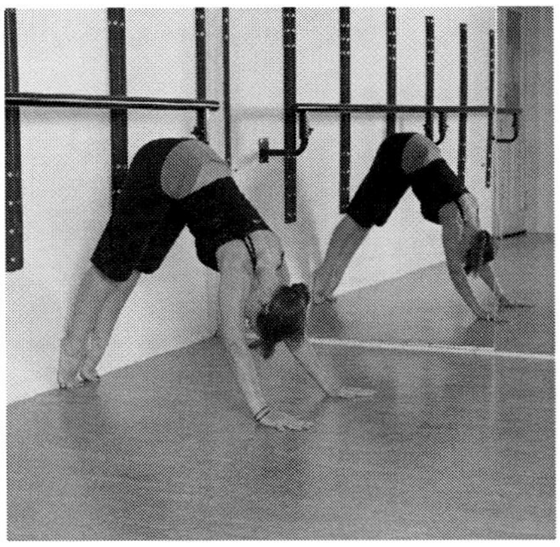

Aim

This exercise strengthens the upper body, whilst stretching the hamstrings

Starting position

Come to a four point kneeling position with the hands under the shoulders and the knees under the hips. The heels are placed against the edge of the wall with the toes tucked under.

Action

Inhale – to prepare

Exhale – to straighten the legs and stick out the buttocks in the air until the body forms and inverted V shape with the elbows and knees straight. This position is held as long as the body is able to maintain good technique. Aim to hold for a minimum of

20 seconds up to 2 minutes breathing normally throughout

Inhale – to bend the knees and return to the starting position

Target Muscles

Deltoids, trapezius, hamstrings

Watchpoints

- Maintain good scapula stability, with ears away from the shoulders
- Keep the hips, shoulders and pelvis as square and stable as possible
- Ensure good, deep breathing throughout
- Try to keep the legs as straight as possible
- The spine should be as flat as possible, depending upon flexibility
- Keep equal weight between the thumb and the little finger
- Keep pushing the rib cage back towards the thighs
- Do not allow the ribs to flare

Variation One (adaptation)

To make this exercise easier, change the starting position. Move the hands forwards so that they are in front of the shoulders (not directly underneath).

Variation Two (progression)

To make this exercise harder, change the starting position. Move the hands back towards the wall so that they are closer to the feet. This makes it more challenging for the upper body and legs

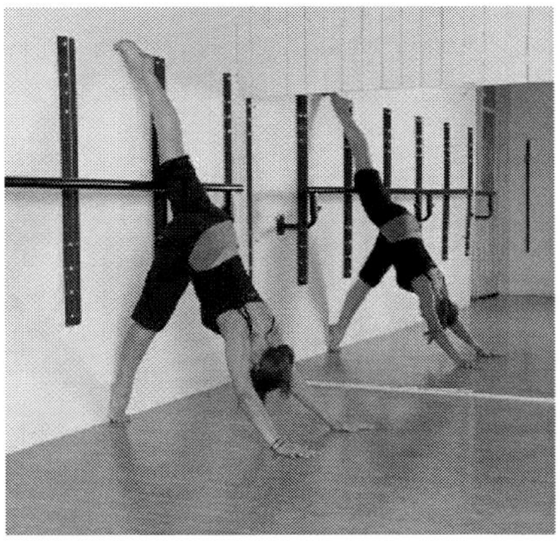

Variation Three

Variation Three (progression)

Adopt the basic V stretch position as before and then lift one leg up in the air against the wall. Walk the hands further in towards the wall to add in a hamstring stretch

Contraindications

This exercise places extra pressure on the wrist joint so may be unsuitable for those with carpal tunnel syndrome or similar wrist problems

Handstand Preparations

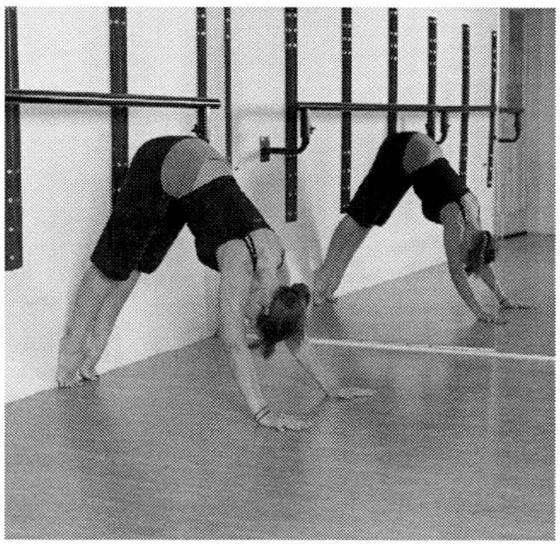

Aim

This is a very challenging exercise, which strengthens the upper body and requires great control and balance

Starting position

Come to a four point kneeling position with the hands under the shoulders and the knees under the hips. The heels are placed against the edge of the wall with the toes tucked under. Straighten the legs and stick out the buttocks in the air until the body forms and inverted V shape with the elbows and knees straight.

Action

Inhale – to prepare

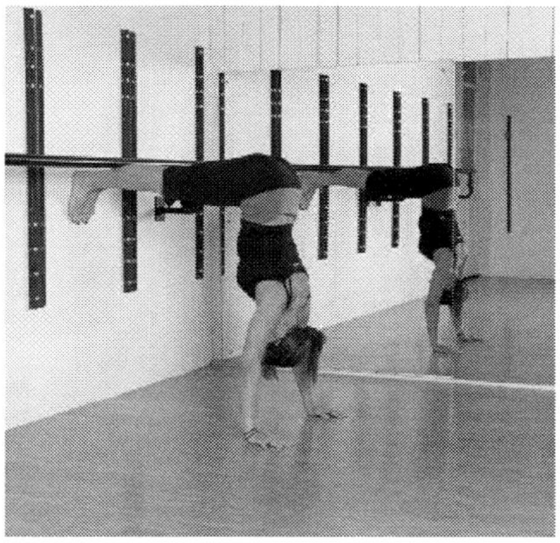

Exhale – To place one foot on the wall just above shoulder height with the knee bent. When the foot is securely in position, lift the second leg off the floor and place the other foot against the wall at the same height with the knee bent. Slowly and gradually aim to straighten the legs, keeping the buttocks roughly in the same position in space. If the legs are straightened and the buttocks move forwards, then the weight comes away from the feet and the legs fall down off the wall. Ideally the body forms a 90 degree angle with the buttocks being directly held over the shoulders and hands (it often feels like you are going to fall over when you are in the correct position so gradually ease the legs straight as it can be a bit daunting initially). This position is held as long as the body is able to maintain good technique. Aim to hold for a minimum of 10-30 seconds breathing normally throughout

Inhale – to bend the knees and place the feet on the floor to return to the starting position

Target Muscles

Deltoids, trapezius

Watchpoints

- Maintain good scapula stability, with ears away from the shoulders
- Keep the hips, shoulders and pelvis as square and stable as possible
- Ensure good, deep breathing throughout
- Try to keep the legs as straight as possible
- The spine should be as flat as possible, depending upon flexibility
- Keep equal weight between the thumb and the little finger
- Keep pushing the rib cage back towards the thighs
- Do not allow the ribs to flare

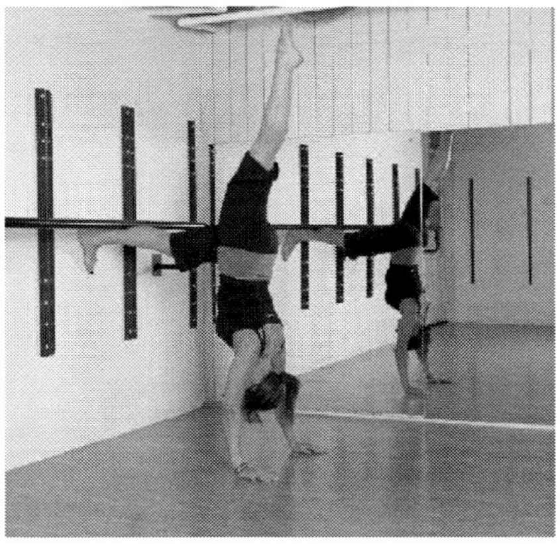

Variation Two

Variation One (adaptation)

To make this exercise easier, change the starting position. Move the hands forwards so that they are in front of the shoulders (the further forwards the hands, the easier the exercise).

Variation Two (progression)

Although this is classed as a progression, since one leg lifts in the air, the work for the upper body is slightly easier. Adopt the basic handstand preparation position as before and then lift one leg in the air. This adds balance as well as a hamstring stretch

Contraindications

This exercise places extra pressure on the wrist joint so may be unsuitable for those with carpal tunnel syndrome or similar wrist problems

Mermaid Stretch

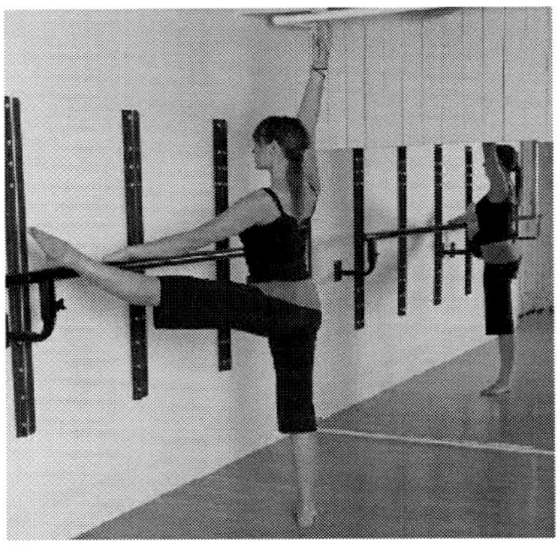

Aim

This exercise stretches the hamstrings, adductors and lateral flexors of the spine

Starting position

Stand upright sideways on to the barre with one hand on the barre and the feet in first position. This stretch may also be done facing the barre (as shown)

Action

Exhale – Place the foot of the leg nearest to the barre onto the top of the barre, maintaining the external rotation of the leg

Inhale – to prepare

Exhale – to raise the free arm up overhead and laterally flex the spine towards the working leg. As the side bend is performed, ensure that the torso remains square and the pelvis level. Repeat with the opposite leg.

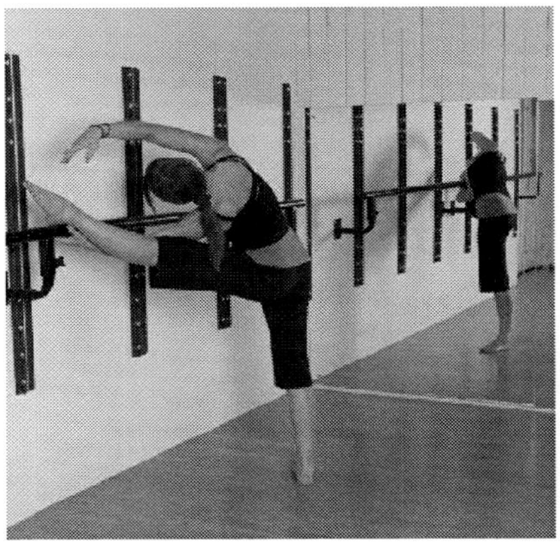

Target Muscles

Adductors, hamstrings, latissimus dorsi, quadratus lumborum

Watchpoints

- Maintain good scapula stability, with ears away from the shoulders
- Ensure the spine does not twist towards the leg when performing the side bend
- Maintain the turnout of the leg in external rotation, particularly when performing the side bend
- If the either the pelvic stability or turnout is lost then the working leg may be moved slightly forwards along the barre so that it is in front of the supporting leg (not level). This position requires less flexibility and therefore a more stable pelvis can be obtained
- Keep the hips, shoulders and pelvis as square and stable as possible with both ASIS's as level as possible throughout
- Ensure the supporting knee is not locked out

Hamstring Stretch

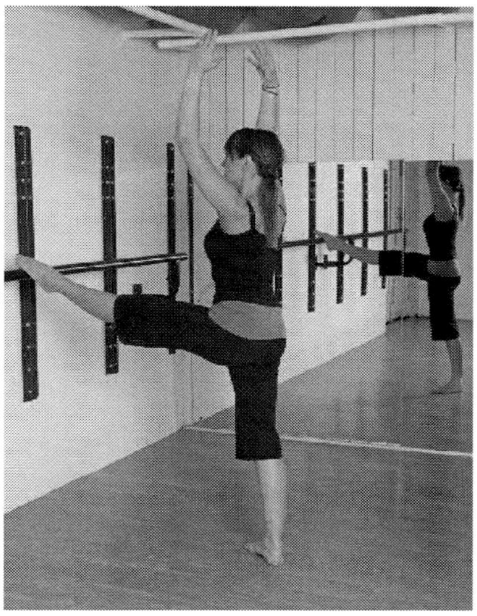

Aim

This exercise stretches the hamstrings

Starting position

Stand upright facing the barre with the feet in a parallel position and both hands on the barre, arms length away

Action

Exhale – Place one foot on the top of the barre, keeping the hips and shoulders square and both legs straight

Inhale – to prepare and raise both arms up in the air

Exhale – to hinge forwards from the waist and bring the arms down to touch the leg as close to the foot as flexibility allows. Repeat with the opposite leg.

Target Muscles

Adductors, hamstrings

Watchpoints

- Maintain good scapula stability, with ears away from the shoulders
- Keep the hips, shoulders and pelvis as square and stable as possible
- Ensure the supporting knee is not locked out

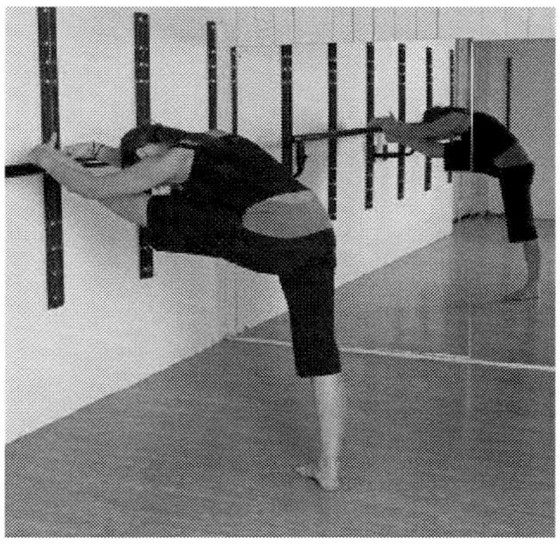

Side Splits

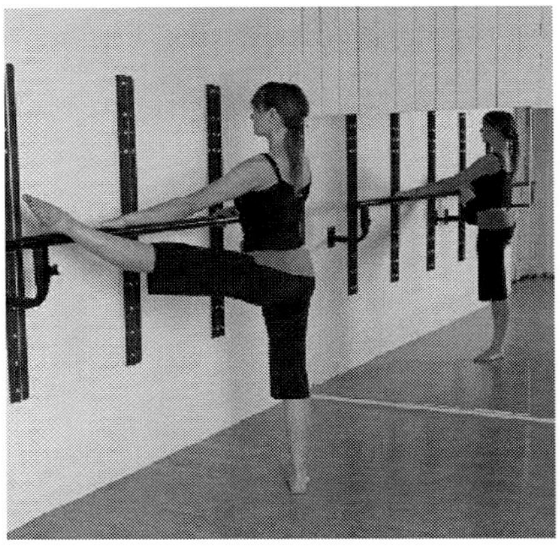

Aim

This exercise stretches the hamstrings and adductors

Starting position

Stand upright facing the barre with the feet in first position and both hands on the barre.

Action

Exhale – Place one foot on the top of the barre, maintaining the external rotation of the leg and keeping the hips and shoulders square

Inhale – to prepare

Exhale – to slide the leg along the barre as far as flexibility allows, whilst maintaining stability in the supporting leg. Repeat with the opposite leg.

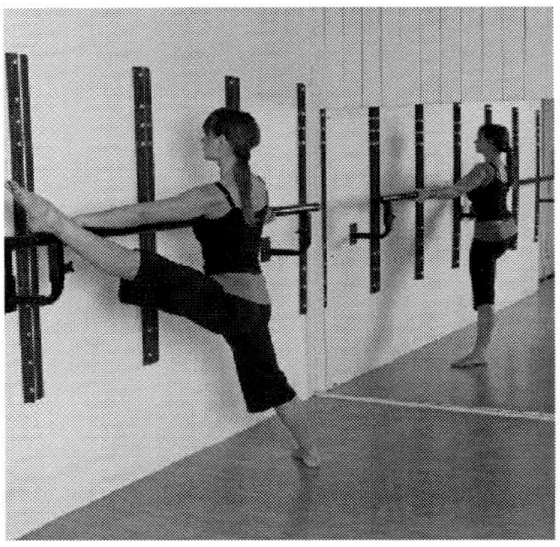

Target Muscles

Adductors, hamstrings

Watchpoints

- Maintain good scapula stability, with ears away from the shoulders
- Maintain the turnout of the leg in external rotation
- Keep the hips, shoulders and pelvis as square and stable as possible
- Ensure the supporting knee is not locked out

Swan Stretch

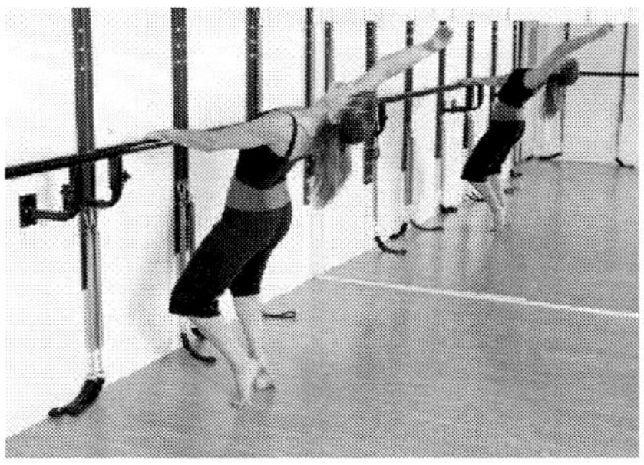

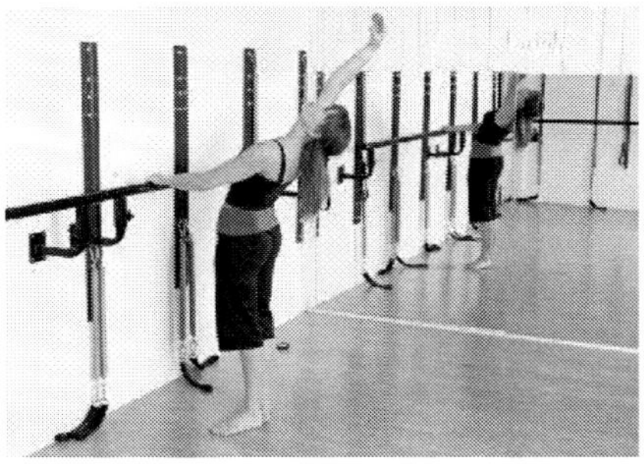

Aim

This exercise stretches the abdominals and mobilises the spine

Starting position

Stand upright facing the barre with the feet in first position and both hands on the barre, arms length away

Action

Inhale – to prepare and raise one arm up in the air

Exhale – to gradually bend backwards as flexibility allows, whilst maintaining a stable pelvis. Repeat with the opposite arm. This may also be performed in a demi plié position.

Target Muscles

Abdominals, spinal extensors

Watchpoints

- Maintain good scapula stability, with ears away from the shoulders
  Keep the hips, shoulders and pelvis as square and stable as possible
- Ensure the neck does not hyperextend
- Try not to pull on the barre whilst performing the back bend
- Ensure the bend comes from the spine and not the hips or legs

Contraindications

This exercise may be unsuitable for certain disc related back problems. The head may be kept in a neutral position if any discomfort is experienced in the cervical spine

Standing Glute Stretch

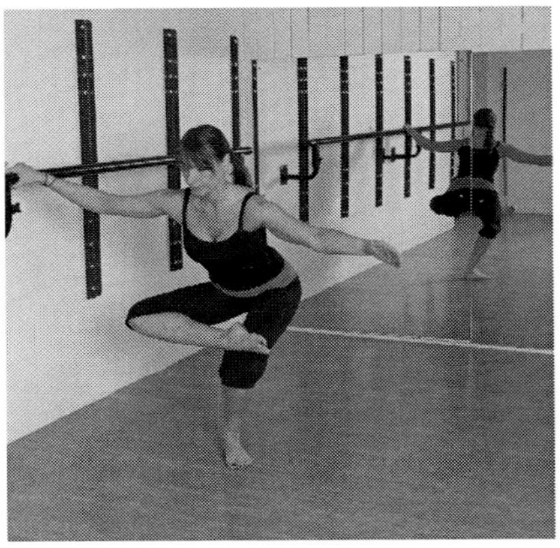

Aim

This exercise stretches the glutes

Starting position

Stand upright sideways on to the barre with the feet in parallel.

Action

Inhale – to prepare

Exhale – to bend the right knee and cross the right ankle over the left thigh. The left knee bends into a demi plié and the torso leans forwards. Aim to open the right knee out to the side as wide as possible. Hold for around 10-20 seconds and repeat on the opposite side.

Target Muscles

Glutes

Watchpoints

- Maintain good scapula stability, with ears away from the shoulders
- Keep the hips, shoulders and pelvis as square and stable as possible. The spine should be in a neutral position whilst leaning forwards
- Ensure the foot that rests on the opposite thigh does not "sickle"

Standing Quad Stretch

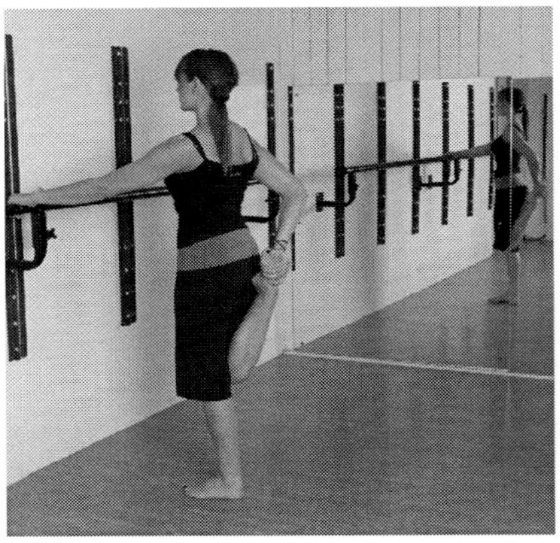

Aim

This exercise stretches the quadriceps

Starting position

Stand upright sideways on to the barre with the feet in parallel.

Action

Inhale – to prepare

Exhale – to bend the right knee and bring the right heel towards the right buttock. Hold for around 10-20 seconds and repeat on the opposite side.

Target Muscles

Quadriceps

Watchpoints

- Maintain good scapula stability, with ears away from the shoulders
- Keep the hips, shoulders and pelvis as square and stable as possible to prevent the buttocks from sticking out and the lumbar spine arching
- Ensure the knees stay level to prevent the knee of the leg that is being stretched moving in front of the other knee. The inner thighs should be active, keeping the legs adducted together.

Standing Hip Flexor Stretch

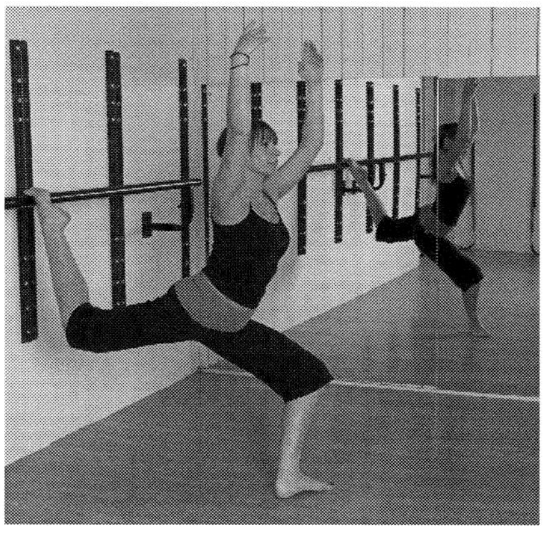

Aim

This exercise stretches the hip flexors

Starting position

Stand upright facing away from the barre with the feet in parallel.

Action

Inhale – to prepare

Exhale – to bend both knees and lift the right leg backwards until the front of the foot is touching the barre. Bend the left knee further for a deeper stretch. Hold for around 10-20 seconds and repeat on the opposite side.

Target Muscles

Iliopsoas

Watchpoints

- Maintain good scapula stability, with ears away from the shoulders
- Keep the hips, shoulders and pelvis as stable as possible
- If the foot cannot reach the barre, this may be performed with the back leg touching the wall lower down

Standing Spinal Twist

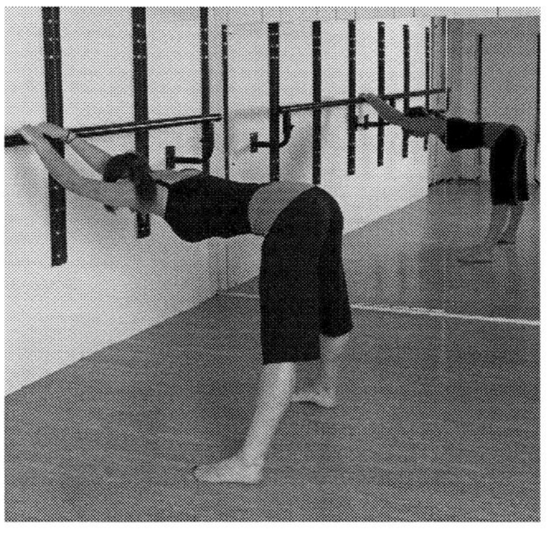

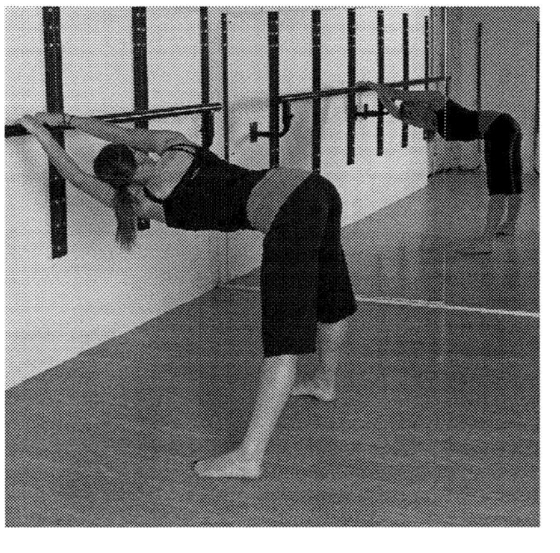

Aim

This exercise stretches and mobilises the spine

Starting position

Stand facing the barre, arms length away, with the feet in parallel and hip width apart. Hinge forwards from the waist and place the hands on the barre, one on top of the other. The back is flat with the spine in a neutral position.

Action

Inhale – to prepare

Exhale – to twist the torso to the right. Look underneath the right armpit. The right shoulder will be higher than the left and the stretch will be felt on the left hand side. Return to the centre and then repeat on the opposite side.

Target Muscles

Lats, obliques, deltoids, hamstrings

Watchpoints

IN THE CENTRE

Resistance Training

Bicep Curls
Tricep Extension Variations
Tummy Rub
The Waiter
Front Shoulder Raise
Lateral Shoulder Raise
Chariot
Back Rowing
Aeroplane
Chest Press
Overhead Press

Motor Skills

Arabesque
Plies with Arabesque
Ballet Jumps in First
Ballet Jumps in Second
Ballet Jumps from First to Second
Échappé Sauté
Changements
Jeté
Standing side leg abduction
Standing back leg raise
Standing front leg raise

Resistance Training

For this section, choose from **weights, toning balls or stretch bands** to provide upper body resistance. We are using weights for this section. Weights should be between 0.5-2 lbs. Repetitions numbers should be around 8-12 and between 1-3 sets are performed. The exercises may be performed in a static standing position in either parallel with legs hip distance apart or in second position in turnout. For a more dynamic, advanced workout, leg movements can be added such as lunges, plies, ronds de jambe and squats to make it more challenging. Balance and strength can be challenged by performing the resistance training with one leg raised out behind the body (as in a low arabesque). Combine movements such as chest press and overhead pree together, rather than separately (e.g. 1 x chest press followed by 1 x overhead press).

Squat with Bicep Curl

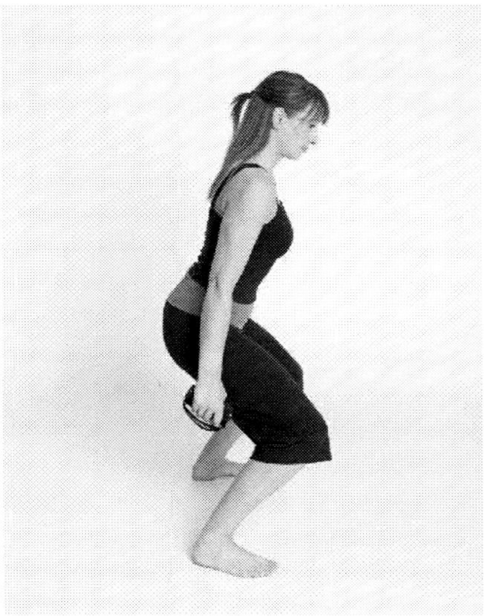

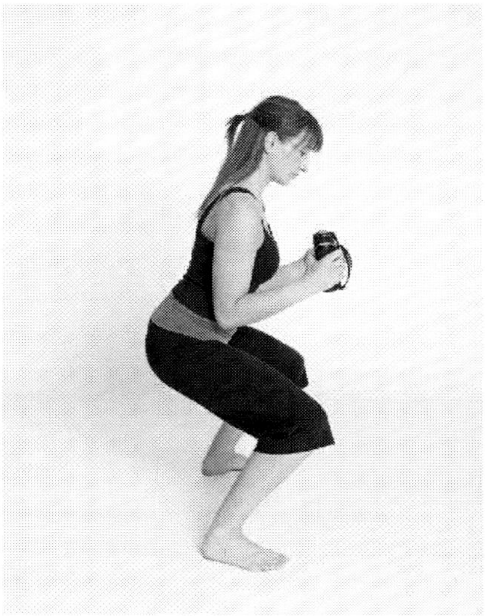

Aim

To strengthen the biceps, glutes and quadriceps and maintain a neutral spine

Starting Position

Stand upright with both feet wider than shoulder width apart. Hold a weight in each hand. The upper arms are down by the sides of the body.

Action

Inhale - to prepare

Exhale – engage the core abdominals and bend the knees and squat down. During the squat, the buttocks stick out behind the shoulders and the torso leans slightly forwards but the spine remains in a neutral position. Simultaneously bend the elbows to perform a bicep curl.

Inhale - to return to the starting position

Watchpoints

- Ensure that the hips do not go below the level of the knee on the squat
- Use the core abdominals well to maintain the spine in a neutral position throughout
- Keep the upper arms glued to the side of the body to ensure that only the forearm moves. The elbows should remain in a fixed position throughout and not move forwards or backwards as the bicep curl is performed.
- Keep the shoulders away from the ears

Variation One (Adaptation)

This exercise may be performed doing single alternate bicep curls rather than lifting two weights at the same time.

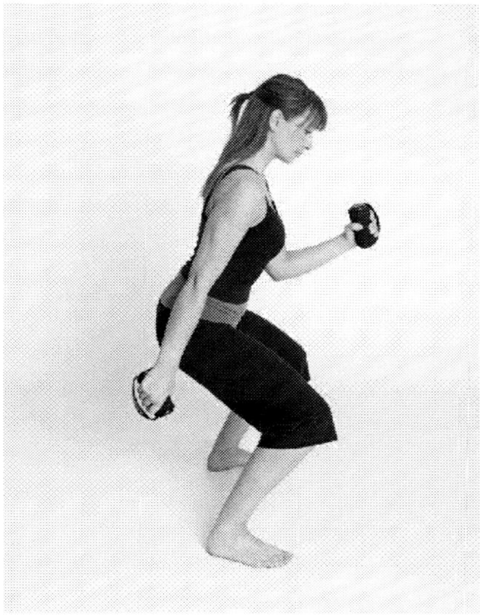

Variation One

Contra-Indications

There is extra stress on the knee joint during a squat. A smaller bend can be performed or if any discomfort is felt then this may be unsuitable.

Tricep Kickback in Front Lunge

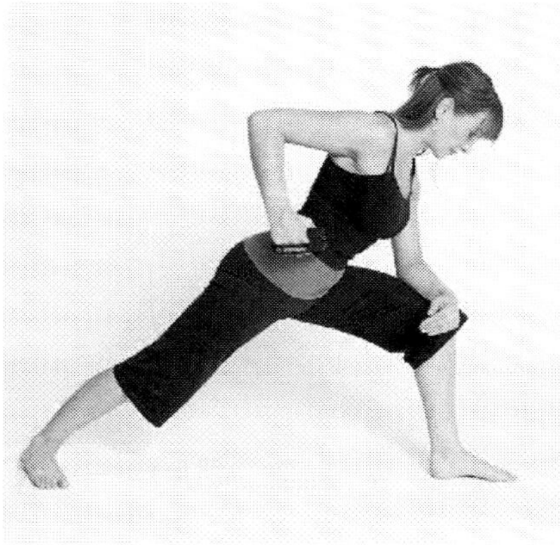

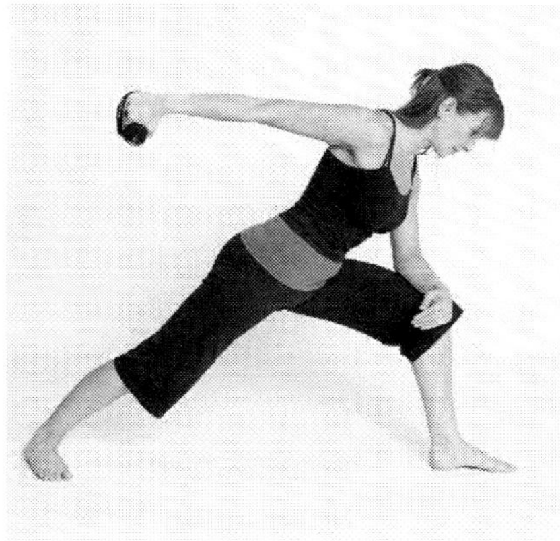

Aim

To strengthen the triceps and quadriceps

Starting Position

Stand upright with the left leg straight back behind the body about two feet away from the right leg. Bend the right knee whilst maintaining a straight left leg so that the body is in a lunge position. The right elbow may rest upon the right thigh to help maintain the position of the torso. Hold a weight in the left hand and bend the left elbow at around 90 degrees until the elbow is at shoulder height, with the hand directly below the elbow. Keep the elbow close in towards the body.

Action

Inhale - to prepare

Exhale - to engage the core abdominals and straighten the elbow backwards behind the body until the hand is level with the shoulder

Inhale - to bend the arm back to the starting position, keeping the elbow in a fixed position

Target Muscles

Triceps

Watchpoints

- Ensure that the shoulders do not hike up to the ears
- Keep the collar bones wide and open
- Maintain core engagement throughout to ensure a neutral spine
- Ensure that the elbow does not drop below the level of the shoulder as it straightens
- Keep the wrist in a neutral alignment

Variation One (Progression)

This exercise may be done with both arms at the same time

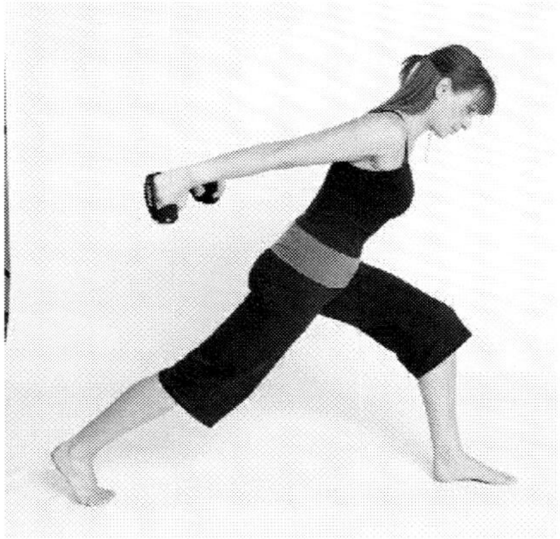

Variation One

Tricep Extension in Side Lunge

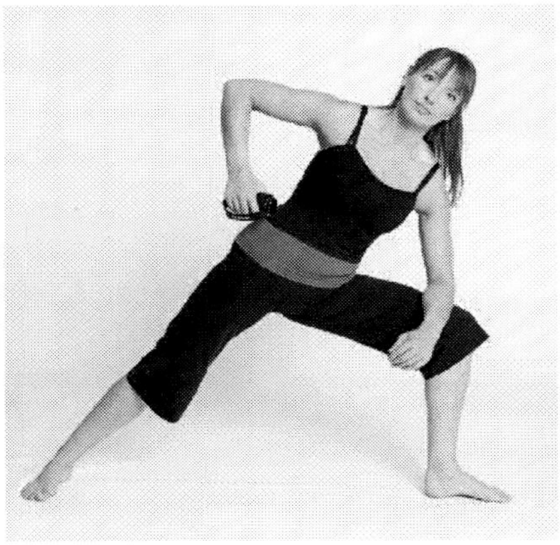

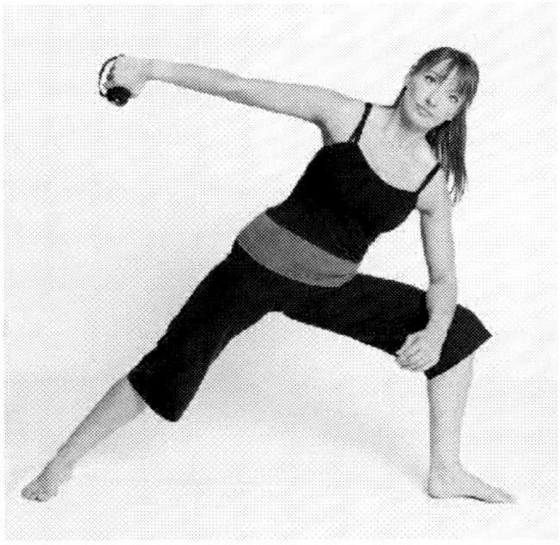

Aim

To strengthen the triceps and quadriceps

Starting Position

Stand upright with the feet wide apart. The right foot is pointing out sideways, whilst the left foot faces directly forwards. Bend the right knee whilst maintaining a straight left leg so that the body is in a side lunge position. Hold the weight in the left hand and bend the left elbow at around 90 degrees until the elbow is around shoulder height, with the hand directly below the elbow

Action

Inhale - to prepare

Exhale - to engage the core abdominals and straighten the elbow directly out to the left side of the body at shoulder height

Inhale - to bend the arm back to the starting position, keeping the elbow in a fixed position

Target Muscles

Triceps

Watchpoints

- Ensure that the shoulders do not hike up to the ears
- Keep the collar bones wide and open
- Maintain core engagement throughout to ensure a neutral spine
- Ensure that the elbow does not drop below the level of the shoulder as it straightens
- Keep the wrist in a neutral alignment

Tummy Rub in Side Lunge

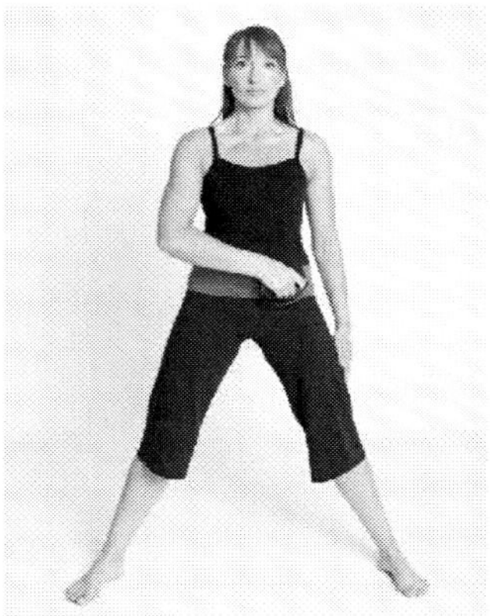

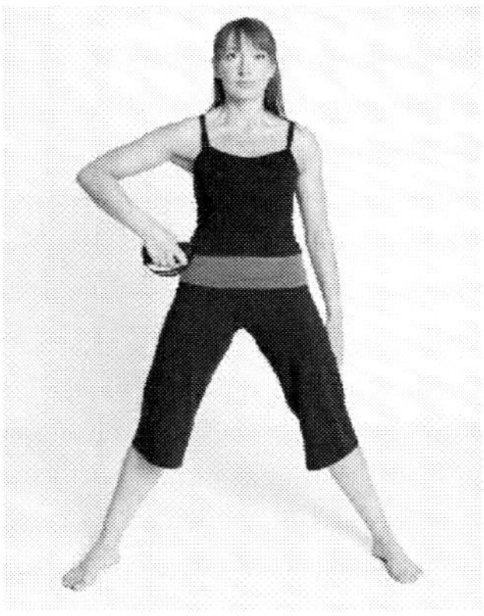

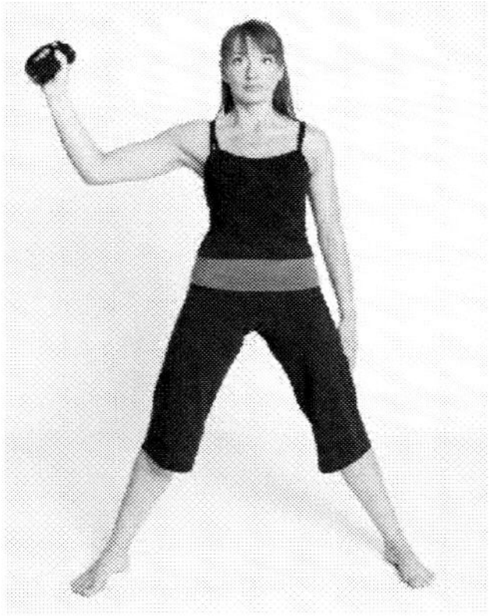

Aim

To work the external and internal rotators of the arm

Starting Position

Stand upright with the feet shoulder width apart. Hold the weight in the left hand. The elbow is bent out to the side with the fist touching the bottom of the right hip. The palm faces inwards towards the body.

Action

Inhale - to engage the core abdominals and "rub the tummy". The left fist travels in a diagonal line from the bottom of the right hip across to the top of the left hip. The fist, elbow and shoulder all remain in the same plane of alignment (i.e. the elbow does not move behind the wrist). The elbow is bent to the side at around 90 degrees

Exhale - maintaining core engagement and also maintaining that same angle at the elbow, externally rotate the arm upwards to the ceiling. As this happens, the elbow remains in the exact same position in space. The fist travels upwards until it is directly above the elbow at 90 degrees

Inhale - to internally rotate the arm back until the fist is resting on the top of the left hip again

Exhale - to 'rub the tummy", bringing the fist across and down to the bottom of the right hip

Target Muscles

External and internal arm rotators

Watchpoints

- Ensure that the shoulders do not hike up to the ears
- Keep the collar bones wide and open
- Maintain core engagement throughout to ensure a neutral spine
- Ensure that the elbow stays in the same position in space as the arm rotates
- Do not change the joint angle at the elbow as the arm rotates (i.e. do not allow the fist to come closer to the shoulder)
- Keep the wrist in a neutral alignment
- Keep an even alignment with the shoulder, elbow and wrist to prevent the elbow from moving back behind the body as you rub the tummy
- Ensure that the body does not twist when externally rotating the arm

Variation One (Progression)

One the arm has externally rotated, it may then straighten fully before bending again and returning to the starting position

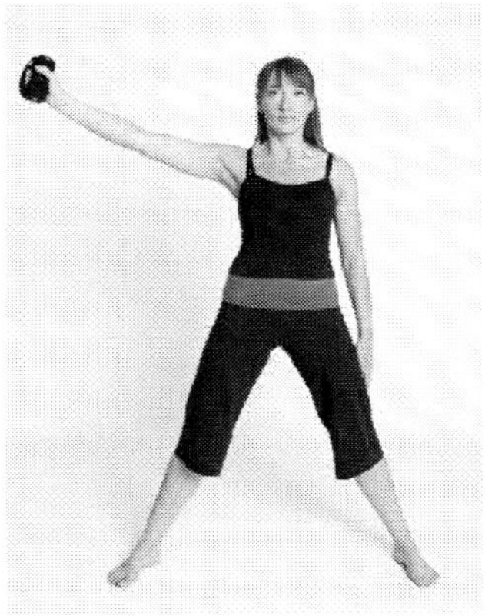

Variation One

The Waiter

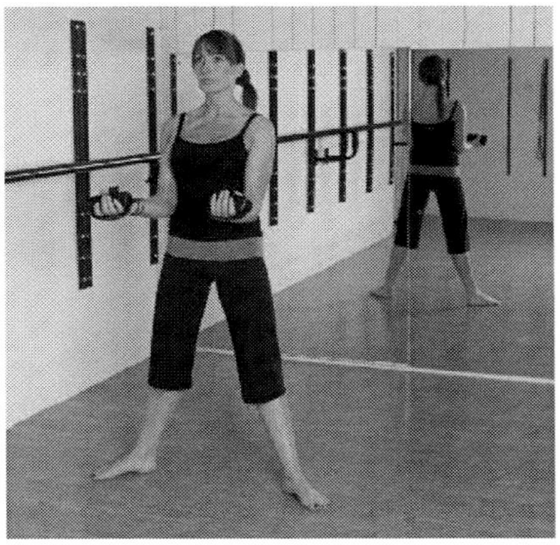

Aim

To learn correct workings and placement of the scapula stabilising muscles

Starting Position

Stand upright with the feet hip width apart. Bend the elbows at a 90 degree angle. The upper arms are glued to the side of the body, whilst the forearms are pointing forwards in front of the body (like a waiter holding a tray). The weight is held in each hand.

Action

Inhale - to prepare

Exhale - to engage the core abdominals and slide the scapula down into the back. Simultaneously open out the forearms to the side. The elbows should endeavour to stay touching the sides of the body and the hands should stay level with the elbows

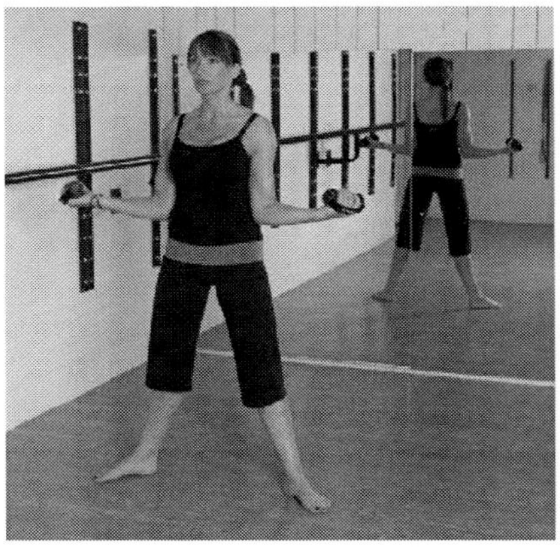

Inhale - to bring the forearms back to the starting position.

Target Muscles

External shoulder rotators

Watchpoints

- As the arms open out, ensure that the ribs do not flare
- Ensure that the shoulders do not hike up to the ears
- Ensure that there is no increase or decrease in the 90 degree angle (i.e. wrists level with the elbows)
- Try to keep the elbows hugging in to the sides of the body throughout
- Keep the wrists in a neutral position throughout

Variation One (Progression)

This exercise may be performed with a plié in second position.

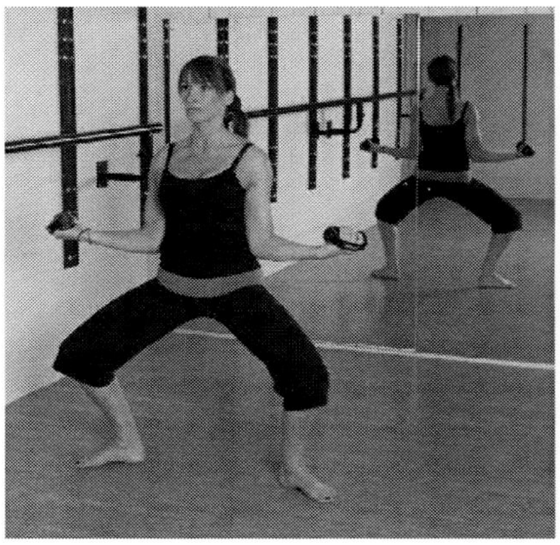

Variation One

Front Shoulder Raise

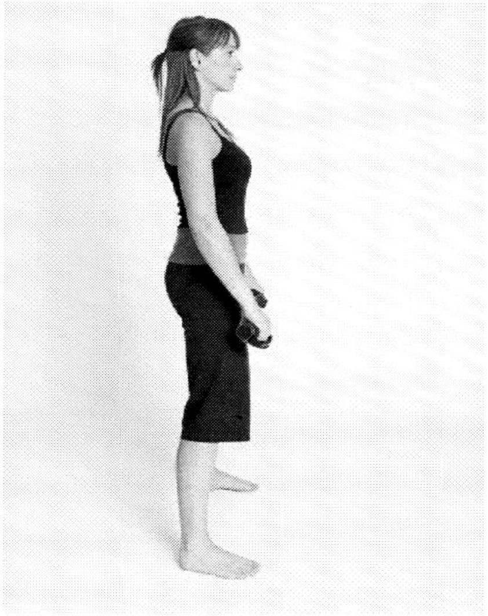

Aim

To work the anterior deltoids, whilst maintaining scapula stability and good posture

Starting Position

Stand upright with the feet wider than shoulder width apart. The arms are straight down by the sides of the body. The palms face the floor as the arms rise up. Hold a weight in each hand.

Action

Inhale - to prepare

Exhale - to engage the core abdominals and raise both arms forwards in front of the body no higher than shoulder level

Inhale - to bring the arms back to the starting position.

Target Muscles

Anterior deltoid, core abdominals

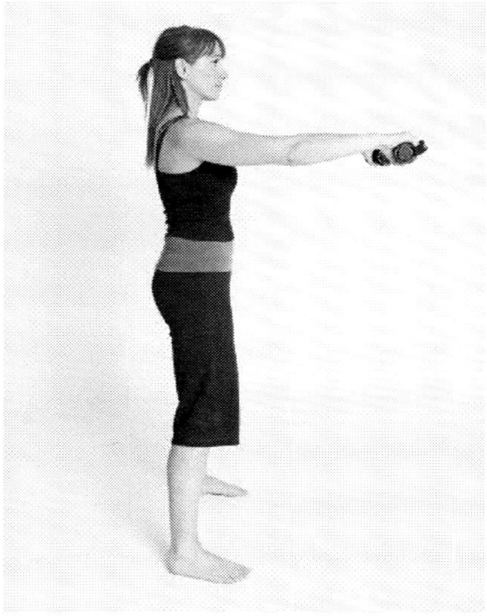

Watchpoints

- As the arms lift, ensure that the body does not lean back
- Ensure that the shoulders do not hike up to the ears
- Keep the collar bones wide and open
- Maintain core engagement throughout to ensure a neutral spine
- Keep the knee joints soft
- Only lift the arms as high as scapula and pelvic stability allow

Variation One (Adaptation)

Instead of lifting both arms together, try lifting one arm at a time and alternate each time.

Lateral Shoulder Raise

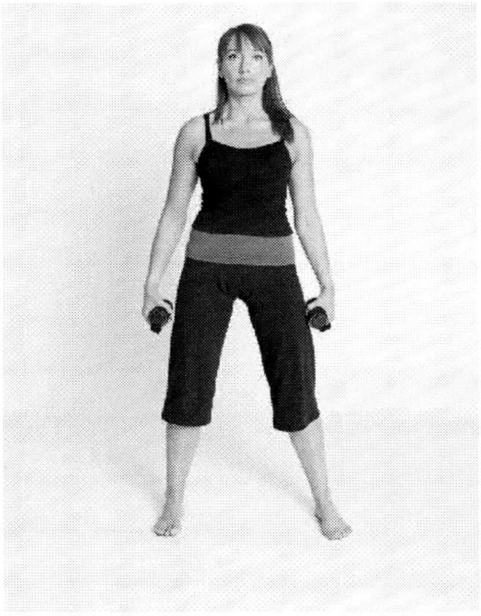

Aim

To work the medial deltoids, whilst maintaining scapula stability and good posture

Starting Position

Stand upright with the feet wider than shoulder width apart. The arms are straight down by the sides of the body. Hold a weight in each hand.

Action

Inhale - to prepare

Exhale - to engage the core abdominals and raise both arms laterally out to the sides of the body no higher than shoulder level. The elbows stay soft and the palms face the floor

Inhale - to bring the arms back to the starting position.

Target Muscles

Medial deltoid, core abdominals

Watchpoints

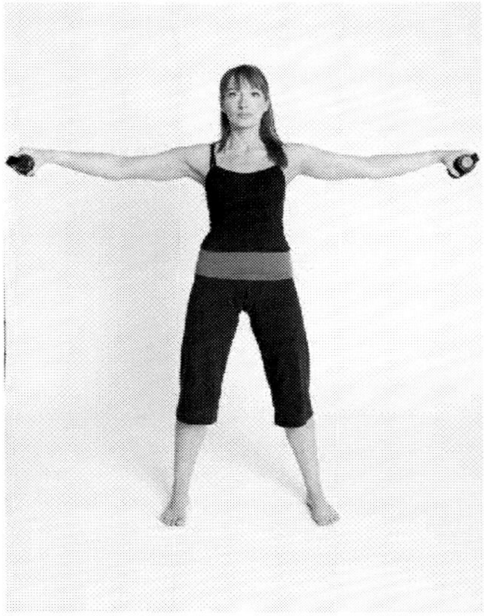

- As the arms lift, ensure that the body does not lean back
- Ensure that the shoulders do not hike up to the ears
- Keep the collar bones wide and open
- Maintain core engagement throughout to ensure a neutral spine
- Keep the knee joints soft
- Only lift the arms as high as scapula and pelvic stability allow

Variation One (Adaptation)

Instead of lifting both arms together, try lifting one arm at a time and alternate each time.

Chariot

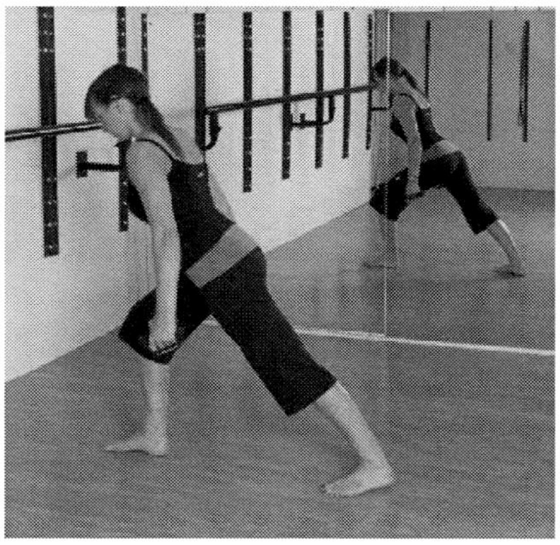

Aim

To open out the chest and strengthen the mid back muscles

Starting Position

Stand upright with one foot forward and the other leg straight back behind the body about two feet away. Bend the front knee whilst maintaining a straight back leg so that the body is in a lunge position. The arms are straight down by the sides of the body. Hold a weight in each hand. The hips and shoulders are square and facing forwards.

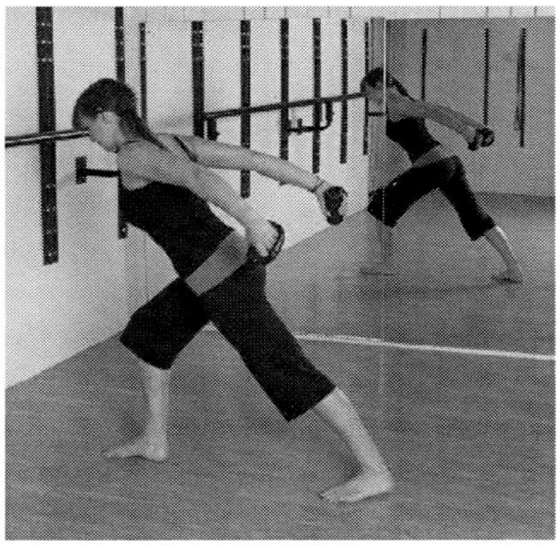

Action

Inhale - to prepare

Exhale - to engage the core abdominals and push both arms backwards behind the body, keeping the elbows straight

Inhale - to bring the arms back to the starting position

Target Muscles

Posterior deltoid, lower trapezius, triceps, core abdominals, rhomboids

Watchpoints

- As the arms pull back, ensure that the body does not also pull back (i.e. keep the front knee bent throughout and the torso slightly leaning forwards)
- Ensure that the shoulders do not hike up to the ears
- Keep the collar bones wide and open
- Maintain core engagement throughout to ensure a neutral spine
- Ensure that the ribs do not flare or the chin poke forwards as the arms pull back
- Keep the elbows soft and the wrists in a neutral alignment

Variation One (Adaptation)

Instead of adopting the lunge position, this exercise may be done standing with both feet level, wider than shoulder width apart.

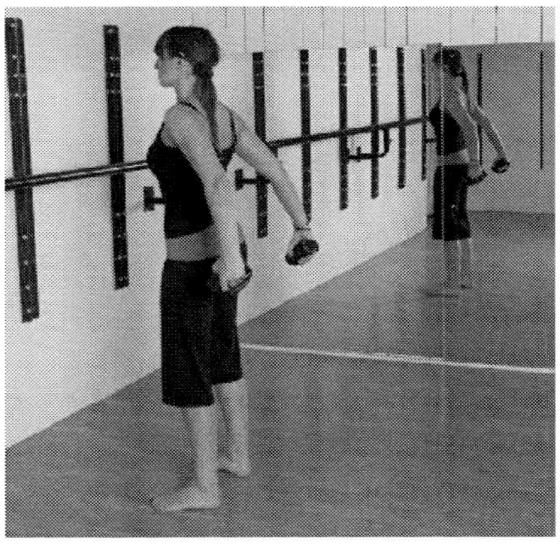

Variation One

Back Rowing

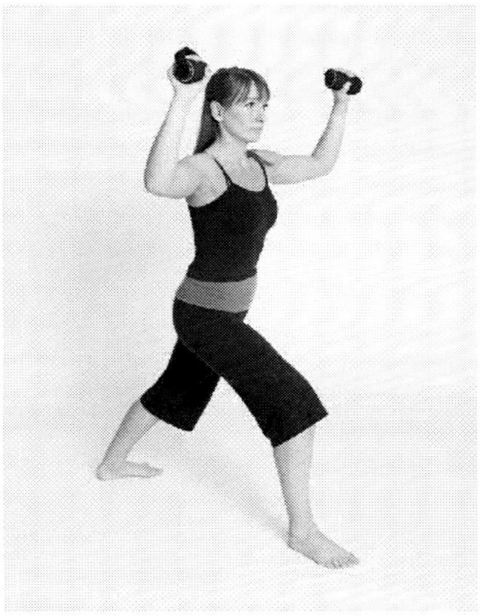

Aim

To open out the chest and strengthen the mid back muscles

Starting Position

Stand upright with leg forwards and the other leg straight back behind the body about two feet away. Bend the front knee whilst maintaining a straight back leg so that the body is in a lunge position. The arms are bent at 90 degrees out to the side. The elbows are at shoulder height and the hands directly above the elbows. Hold a weight in each hand.

Action

Inhale - to prepare

Exhale - to engage the core abdominals and push both arms backwards behind the body, maintaining the 90 degree angle

Inhale - to bring the arms back to the starting position.

Target Muscles

Posterior deltoid, lower trapezius, rhomboids

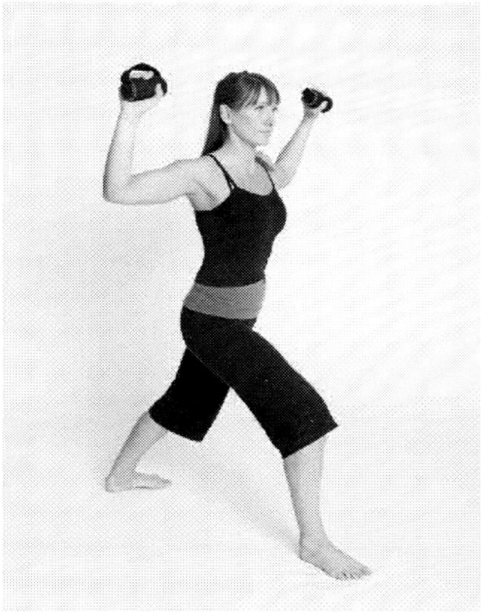

Watchpoints

- As the arms pull back, ensure that the body does not also pull back
- Ensure that the shoulders do not hike up to the ears
- Keep the collar bones wide and open
- Maintain core engagement throughout to ensure a neutral spine
- Ensure that the ribs do not flare or the chin poke forwards as the arms pull back
- Try to keep the elbows at shoulder height throughout

Variation One (Adaptation)

Instead of adopting the lunge position, this exercise may be done standing with both feet level, wider than shoulder width apart.

Aeroplane

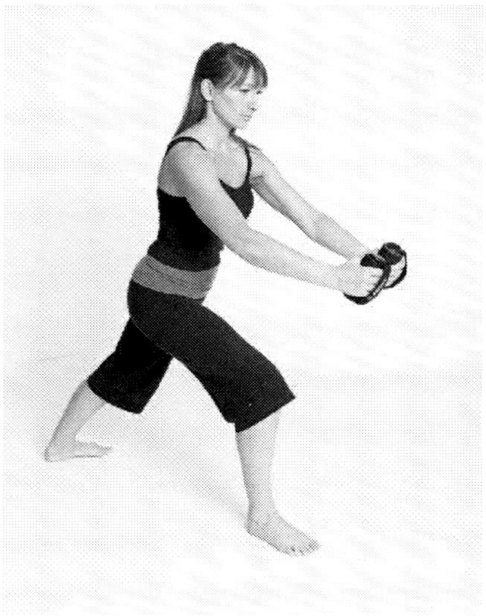

Aim

To open out the chest and strengthen the mid back muscles

Starting Position

Stand upright with one leg forwards and the other leg straight back behind the body about two feet away. Bend the front knee whilst maintaining a straight back leg so that the body is in a lunge position. The arms are extended straight out in front of the chest at shoulder height. Hold a weight in each hand.

Action

Inhale - to prepare

Exhale - to engage the core abdominals and push both arms out to the side and backwards, trying to keep the hands level with the shoulders

Inhale - to bring the arms back to the starting position.

Target Muscles

Posterior deltoid, lower trapezius, triceps, rhomboids

Watchpoints

- As the arms pull back, ensure that the body does not also pull back
- Ensure that the shoulders do not hike up to the ears
- Keep the collar bones wide and open
- Maintain core engagement throughout to ensure a neutral spine
- Ensure that the ribs do not flare or the chin poke forwards as the arms pull back
- Keep the elbows soft and the wrists in a neutral alignment
- Ensure that the scapula do not nip together

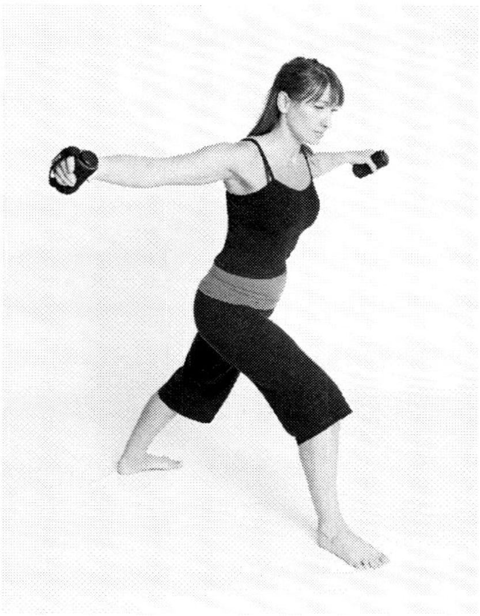

Variation One (Adaptation)

Instead of adopting the lunge position, this exercise may be done standing with both feet level, wider than shoulder width apart.

Chest Press

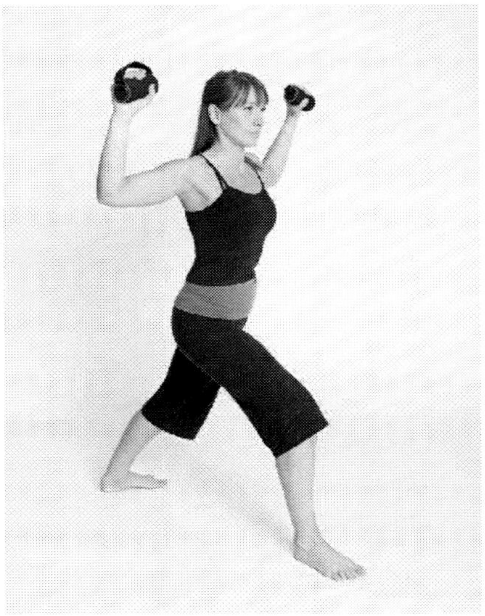

Aim

To strengthen the chest and shoulders

Starting Position

Stand upright with the back foot in a lunge position. The back leg is straight back behind the body about two feet away. Bend the front knee whilst maintaining a straight back leg. The arms are bent at 90 degrees out to the side. The elbows are at shoulder height and the hands directly above the elbows. Hold a weight in each hand.

Action

Inhale - to prepare

Exhale - to engage the core abdominals and pull both arms forwards in front the body, maintaining the 90 degree angle. The arms come together but do not touch. The elbows should be in line with the shoulders as the arms are brought forwards

Inhale - to bring the arms back to the starting position.

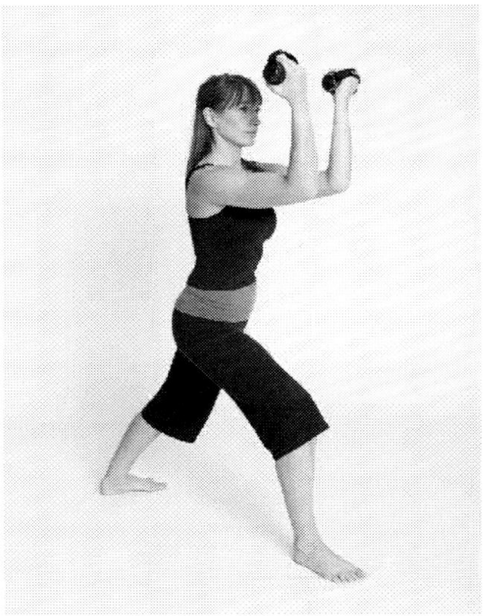

Target Muscles

Pectorals, anterior deltoid

Watchpoints

- As the arms pull forwards, maintain the 90 degree angle at the elbows
- Ensure that the shoulders do not hike up to the ears
- Maintain core engagement throughout to ensure a neutral spine
- Ensure that the arms do not come too close – maintain length in between the two collar bones
- Try to keep the elbows at shoulder height throughout

Variation One (Adaptation)

This exercise may be performed with a lunge or a plié in second position.

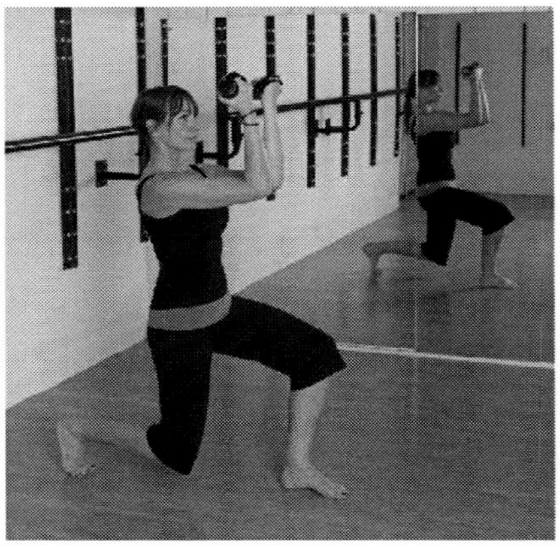

Variation One

Overhead Shoulder Press

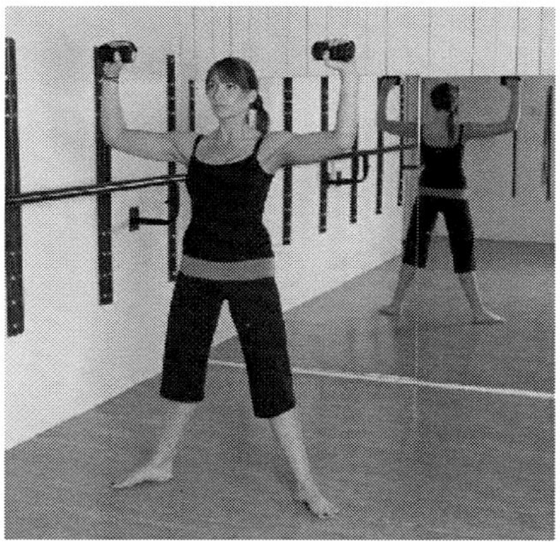

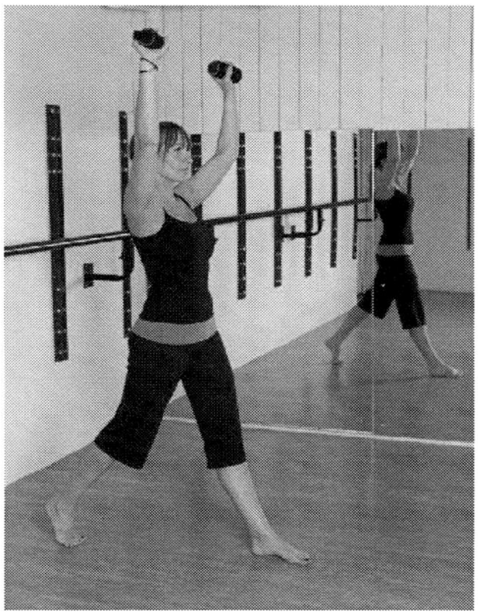

Aim

To strengthen the shoulders whilst maintaining scapula stability

Starting Position

Stand upright with both feet shoulder width apart. The arms are bent at 90 degrees out to the side. The elbows are at shoulder height and the hands directly above the elbows. Hold a weight in each hand.

Action

Inhale - to prepare

Exhale - to engage the core abdominals and push both arms upwards towards the ceiling, straightening the arms as far as scapula stability allows

Inhale - to bring the arms back to the starting position.

Target Muscles

Deltoid, scapula stabilisers

Watchpoints

- Maintain core engagement throughout to ensure a neutral spine
- Ensure that the arms do not come too close together as this will encourage shoulder hiking– maintain length in between the two collar bones and ensure good scapula stability
- Do not lock out the knees when pushing the arms upwards
- Ensure that the ribs do not flare as the elbows straighten
- Keep the back of the neck long and the chin parallel to the floor

Variation One (Progression)

This exercise may be performed in a lunge or a plié in second position

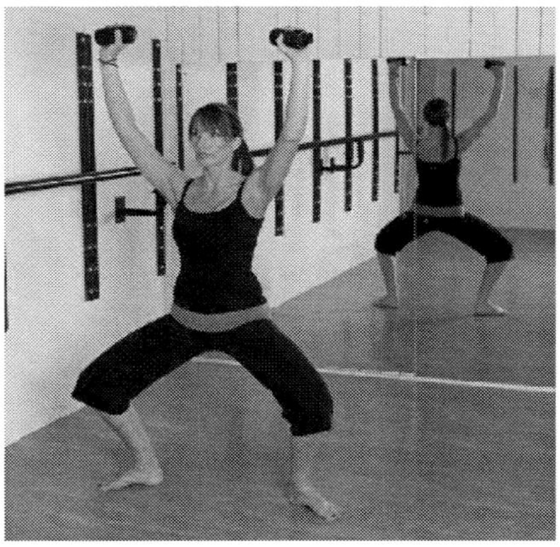

Variation One

In the Centre

Arabesque

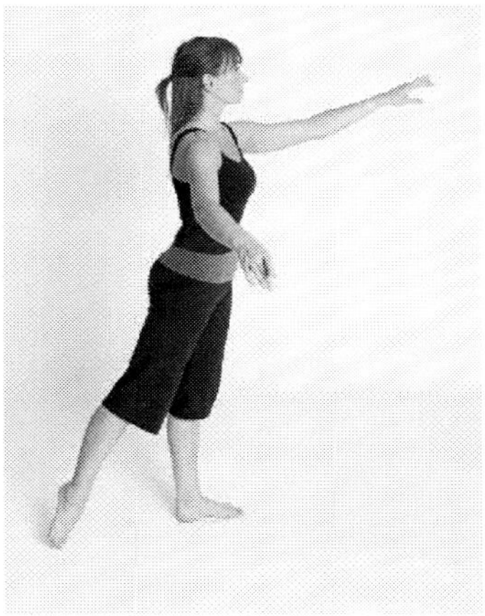

Aim

To increase motor control, balance and co-ordination. This is one of the basic poses in ballet: standing on one leg (which may be straight or in a demi-plié), whilst the other leg is held up behind at right angles to it. The shoulders are square and the arm opposite to the working leg is held forwards, whilst the other arm is held at the side (there are other arm variations) to form a long line with the leg.

Starting Position

Stand upright in first position with the arms in bras bas.

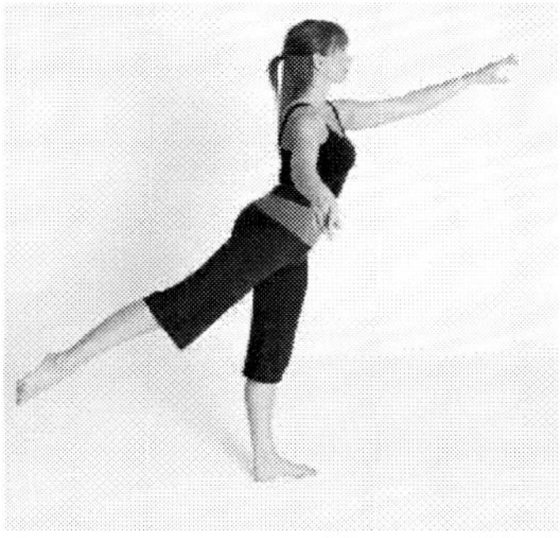

Action

Degagé the right leg off the floor and lift it straight out behind the body as high as possible, maintaining balance. Simultaneously stretch the left arm straight forwards in front at shoulder height, whilst the right arm stretches out to the side at shoulder height. You may want to attempt this exercise close to a wall so that you can put your hands on the wall to help you initially. Try to balance for as long as possible, breathing normally throughout.

Target Muscles

Hamstrings, glutes, quadriceps, gastrocnemus, peroneals, erector spinae, external rotators

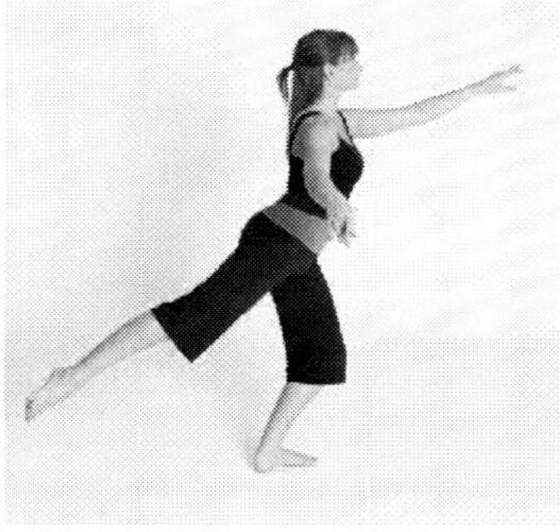

Variation One

Watchpoints

- It may be prudent initially to perform this exercise close to the wall until balance has been established
- Try to keep the waist long on both sides
- Keep the shoulders away from the ears and the neck long
- Do not lock out the knees
- Try to maintain an upright torso as the leg lifts

Variation One (Adaptation)

Hold the arabesque for longer and add in a demi plié on the supporting leg.

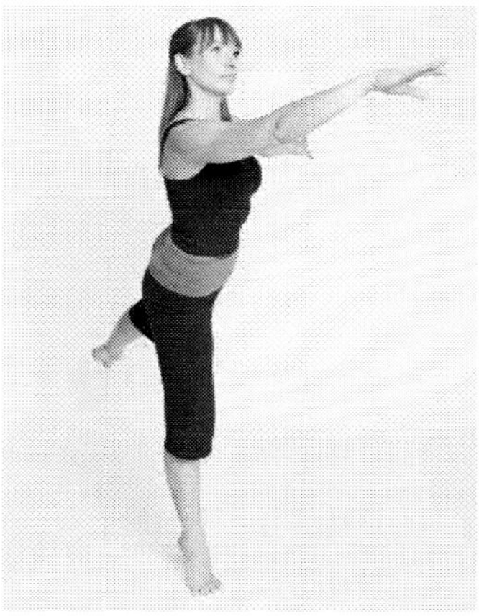

Variation Two

Variation Two (Progression)

A further balance challenge may be added by rising up onto demi pointe on the supporting leg.

Variation Three (Progression)

Penche exercise. Lean forwards towards the floor, maintaining the arabesque position (like a see saw)

Contra-Indications

Avoid initially if any recent foot injuries such as sprained ankles are still present. The combination of maintaining an upright torso, whilst raising the back leg high will put the lumbar spine into extension, which may be uncomfortable for certain back problems. The turned out position of the leg may be unsuitable for sciatica.

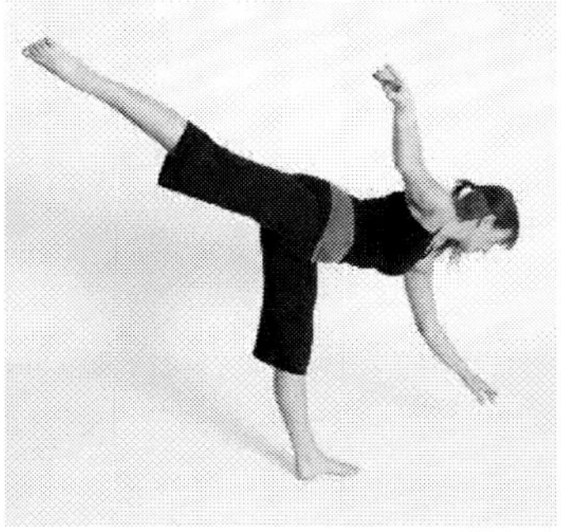

Variation Three

Plié with Arabesque

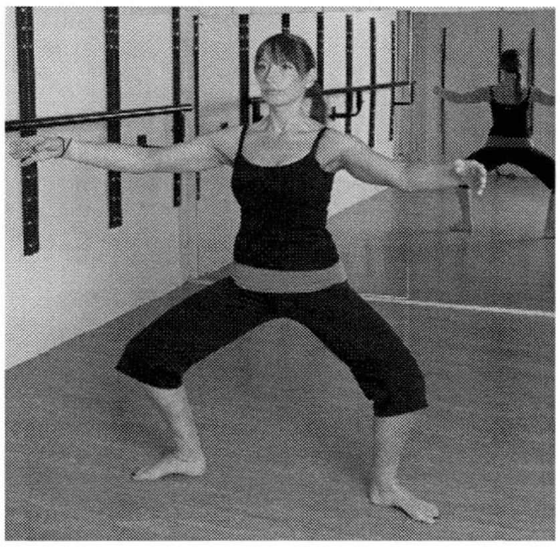

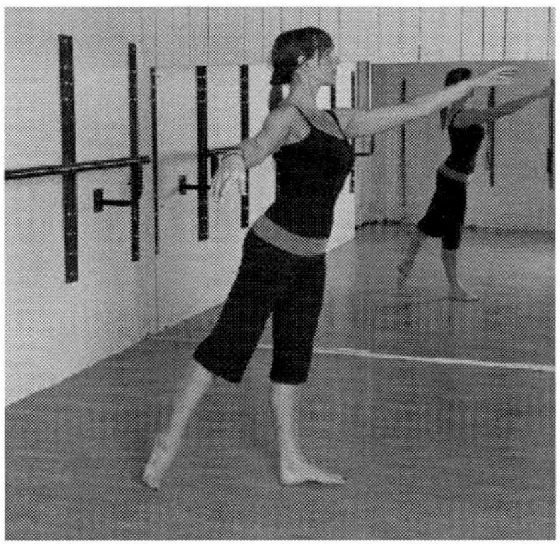

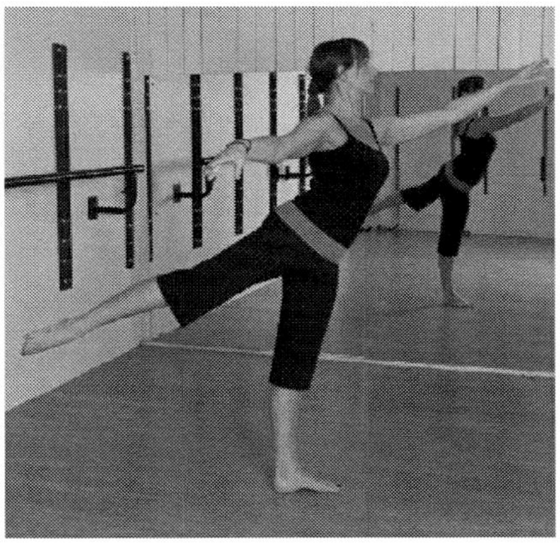

Aim

To strengthen the abductors, glutes and quadriceps and maintain a neutral spine during motion

Starting Position

Stand upright with the feet in Second position and the arms in bras bas.

Action

Inhale - to engage the core abdominals and bend the knees into a grand plié in Second position. Simultaneously bring the arms into Second position

Exhale - straighten the legs and transfer the body weight over to the right leg. Continue exhaling and lift the left leg off the floor into an arabesque

Inhale - to return the foot to the floor and bend the knees into a grand plié in Second position

Exhale - to repeat to the opposite side. Aim for around 8 repetitions to each side

Target Muscles

Hamstrings, glutes, quadriceps, gastrocnemus, soleus, peroneals, erector spinae, external rotators

Watchpoints

- Ensure that the hips do not go below the level of the knee on the plié
- As the leg lifts out into arabesque, ensure that an upright posture is maintained
- Keep the shoulders away from the ears

Variation One (Adaptation)

Leave out the arabesque and just perform the plié with a small transfer of weight onto one leg, without actually raising the foot off the floor.

Variation Two (Progression)

Hold the arabesque for longer and add in a demi plié on the supporting leg. A further balance challenge may be added by rising up onto demi pointe on the supporting leg.

Contra-Indications

There is extra stress on the knee joint during a plié. A smaller bend can be performed or if any discomfort is felt then this may be unsuitable. To avoid excessive lumbar extension, the working leg may be kept at a low height. The turned out position of the leg may be unsuitable for sciatica.

Sauté - Ballet Jump Variations

All ballet jumps involve the tips of the toes being the first to reach the ground after a jump, followed by the sole of the foot and finally, the heel. This order is reversed when rising from the ground. Jumps are best avoided for those with knee problems or substituted with a plié and a relevé instead. These are the first power (strength plus speed) movements involved during an exercise.

Jumps in First Position

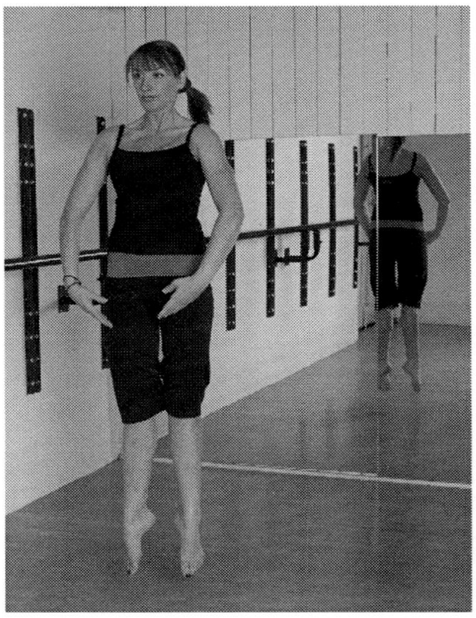

Aim

To strengthen the calves, glutes and quadriceps, whilst maintaining a neutral spine during motion and to increase cardiovascular efficiency and stamina

Starting Position

Stand upright with the feet in First position and the arms in bras bas.

Action

Inhale - to engage the core abdominals and bend the knees into a demi plié. The arms may be held in bras bas or lifted to First position

Exhale – jump quickly into the air, straightening the legs, whilst keeping them adducted and turned out. The toes are stretched into a pointed position

Inhale - to land on the floor gracefully and bend the knees into a demi plié in First position once again before straightening the legs. Aim for up to 10 repetitions

Target Muscles

Hamstrings, glutes, quadriceps, gastrocnemus, peroneals, external rotators

Watchpoints

- Ensure the tips of the toes are the first to reach the ground after the jump, followed by the sole of the foot and then the heel. This order is reversed when rising from the ground.
- Keep the shoulders away from the ears
- Keep the legs adducted when in the air and fully pull up the knee caps
- Land softly and gracefully and allow the petit plié to break the impact
- Keep an upright, neutral spine

Variation One (Adaptation)

Leave out the jump and just perform the plié with a small relevé without the feet actually leaving the floor.

Contra-Indications

There is extra stress on the knee joint during a sauté and this exercise is best avoided if there are any knee or ankle joint problems.

Jumps in Second Position

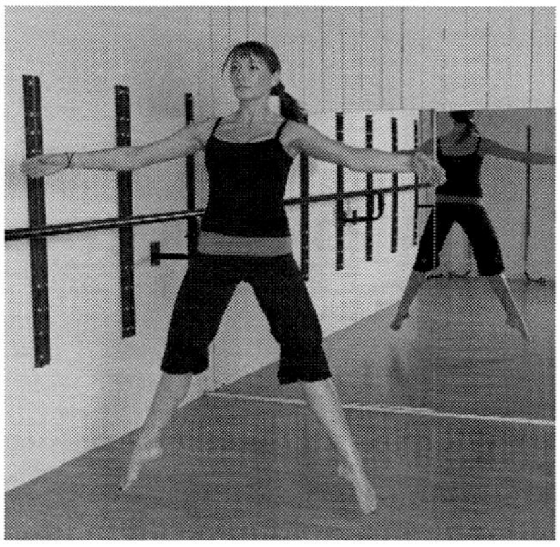

Aim

To strengthen the calves, glutes and quadriceps, whilst maintaining a neutral spine during motion and to increase cardiovascular efficiency and stamina

Starting Position

Stand upright with the feet in Second position and the arms in bras bas.

Action

Inhale - to engage the core abdominals and bend the knees into a demi plié. The arms may be held in bras bas or lifted to Second position

Exhale – jump quickly into the air, straightening the legs, whilst keeping them turned out. The toes are stretched into a pointed position

Inhale - to land on the floor gracefully and bend the knees into a demi plié in Second position once again before straightening the legs. Aim for up to 10 repetitions

Target Muscles

Hamstrings, glutes, quadriceps, gastrocnemus, peroneals, external rotators

Watchpoints

- Ensure the tips of the toes are the first to reach the ground after the jump, followed by the sole of the foot and then the heel. This order is reversed when rising from the ground.
- Keep the shoulders away from the ears
- Keep the legs adducted when in the air and fully pull up the knee caps
- Land softly and gracefully and allow the petit plié to break the impact
- Keep an upright, neutral spine

Variation One (Adaptation)

Leave out the jump and just perform the plié with a small relevé without the feet actually leaving the floor.

Contra-Indications

There is extra stress on the knee joint during a sauté and this exercise is best avoided if there are any knee or ankle joint problems.

Échappé Sauté (Escape) – Jumps from First to Second Position

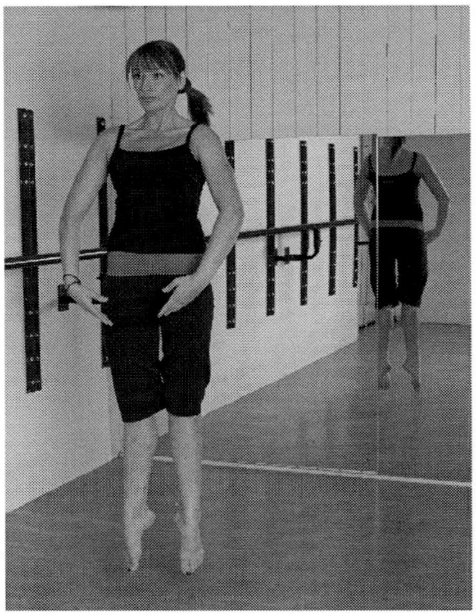

Aim

To strengthen the calves, glutes and quadriceps, whilst maintaining a neutral spine during motion and to increase cardiovascular efficiency and stamina

Starting Position

Stand upright with the feet in First (or fifth) position and the arms in bras bas.

Action

Inhale - to engage the core abdominals and bend the knees into a demi plié and raise the arms to Second position

Exhale – jump quickly into the air, straightening the legs, whilst opening them out into Second position. The toes are stretched into a pointed position

Inhale - to land on the floor gracefully and bend the knees into a demi plié in Second position

Exhale – jump back quickly into the air, straightening the legs, whilst closing them back into First position again. Aim for up to 10 repetitions

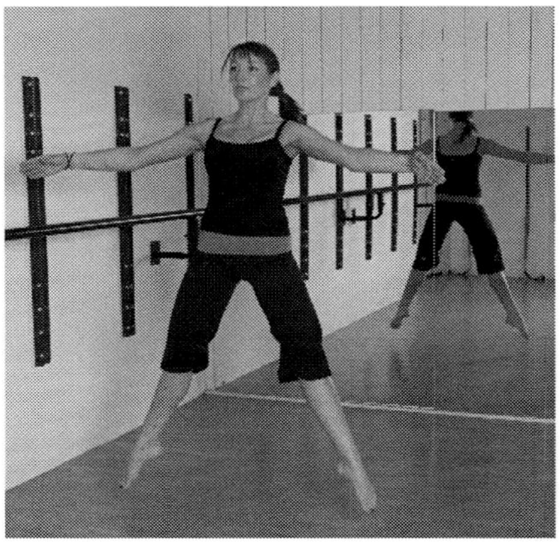

Target Muscles

Hamstrings, glutes, quadriceps, gastrocnemus, peroneals, external rotators

Watchpoints

- Ensure the tips of the toes are the first to reach the ground after the jump, followed by the sole of the foot and then the heel. This order is reversed when rising from the ground.
- Keep the shoulders away from the ears
- Land softly and gracefully and allow the petit plié to break the impact
- Keep an upright, neutral spine
- Ensure both feet jump an equal distance from the centre of gravity

Variation One (Adaptation)

Leave out the jump and just perform the echappé into Second and back again

Contra-Indications

There is extra stress on the knee joint during a sauté and this exercise is best avoided if there are any knee or ankle joint problems.

Changements

Aim

Changements involve the changing of the feet in the air during the jump and it is therefore a little more challenging

Starting Position

Stand upright with the feet in Fifth position, right foot crossed in front, and the arms in bras bas.

Action

Inhale - to engage the core abdominals and bend the knees into a demi plié. The arms may be held in bras bas or lifted to First or Fifth position

Exhale – jump into the air, straightening the legs, and quickly change legs so that the left leg is now crossed in front. The toes are stretched into a pointed position

Inhale - to land on the floor gracefully and bend the knees into a demi plié in Fifth position once again before straightening the legs. The left leg will now be crossed in front. Repeat again and land with the right leg crossed in front once again. Aim for up to 10 repetitions

Target Muscles

Hamstrings, glutes, quadriceps, gastrocnemus, peroneals, external rotators

Watchpoints

- Ensure the tips of the toes are the first to reach the ground after the jump, followed by the sole of the foot and then the heel. This order is reversed when rising from the ground.
- Keep the shoulders away from the ears
- Keep the legs adducted when in the air and fully pull up the knee caps
- Land softly and gracefully and allow the petit plié to break the impact
- Keep an upright, neutral spine

Variation One (Adaptation)

Leave out the jump and just perform the plié with a small relevé without the feet actually leaving the floor.

Contra-Indications

There is extra stress on the knee joint during a sauté and this exercise is best avoided if there are any knee or ankle joint problems.

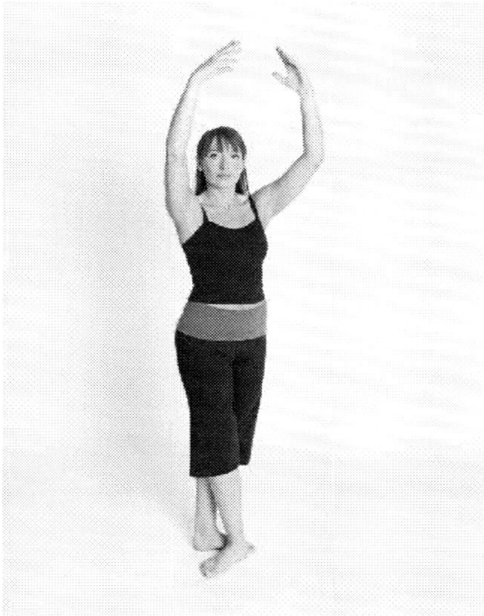

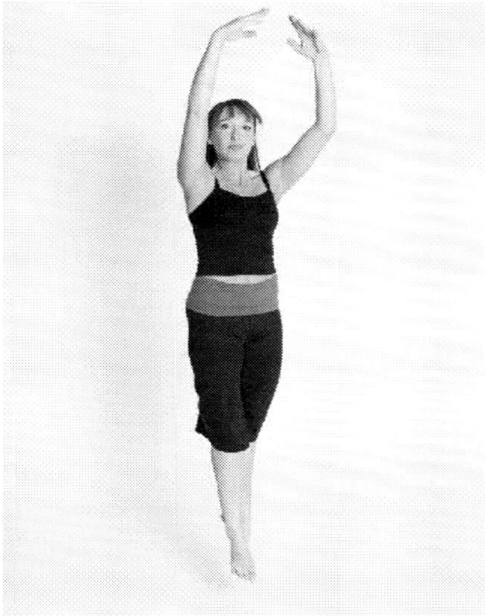

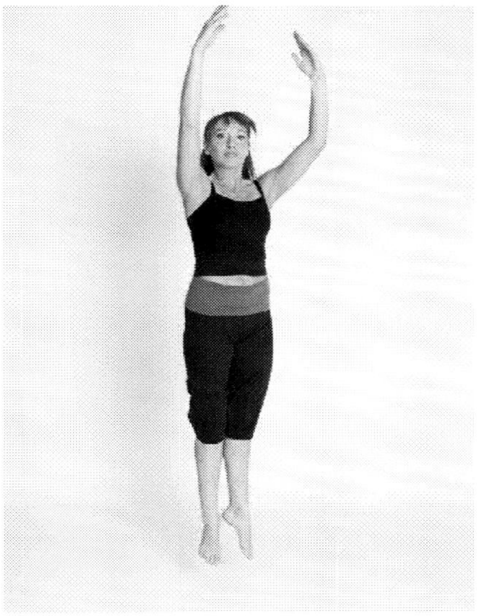

Jeté (Throw)

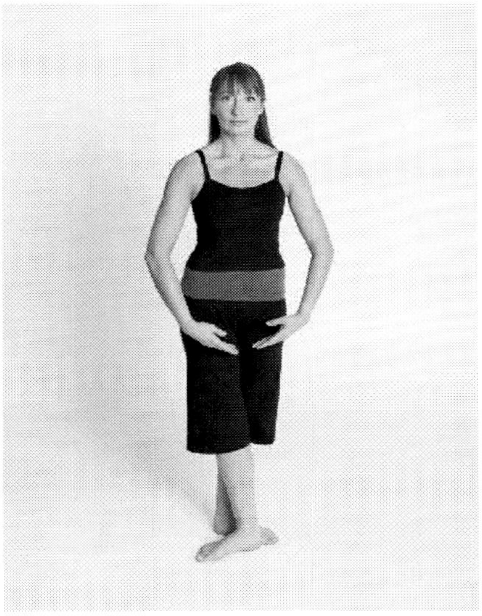

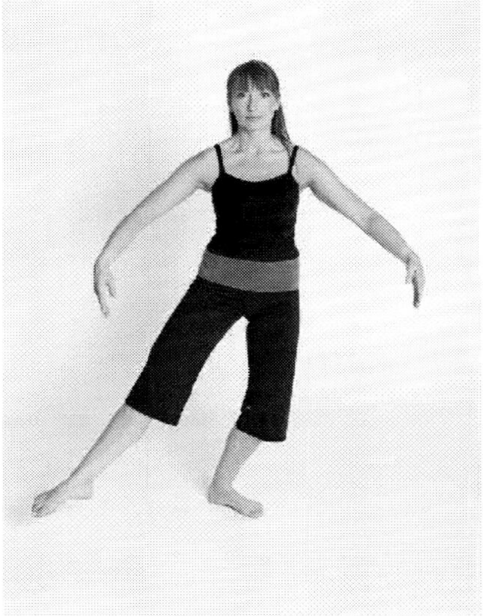

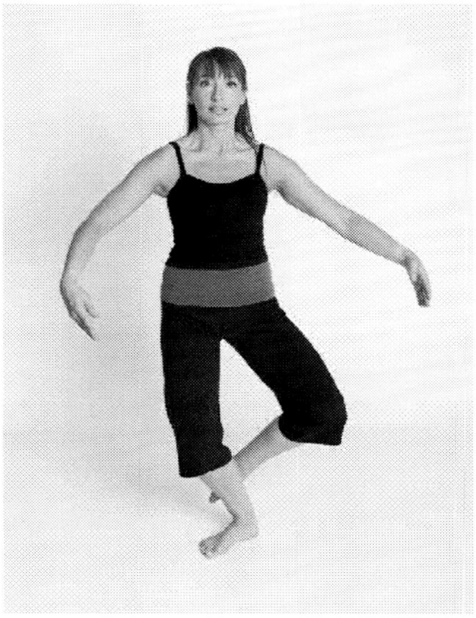

Aim

This involves jumping from one foot to the other. There are many Jetés in ballet but we use a simple variation here. Landing with the impact on one leg only places great stress on the knee joint and this exercise should therefore be used with caution.

Starting Position

Stand upright with the feet in Fifth position and the arms in bras bas.

Action

Inhale - to engage the core abdominals and bend the knees into a demi plié. The arms may be held in bras bas or lifted to First/ Second position

Exhale – degage/ glisse the right leg out to second position, whilst simultaneously jumping into the air

Inhale - to land on the floor gracefully on the right leg and bend both knees into a demi plié. The left leg will also have to bend in order to keep the foot off the floor

Exhale – spring quickly into the air from the right leg and degage/ glisse the left leg out to second position, whilst simultaneously jumping into the air

Inhale – to land on the floor gracefully on the left leg this time and bend the knees into a demi plié. The right leg will also have to bend in order to keep the foot off the floor. Alternate jumping from one leg to another. Aim for up to 10 repetitions

Target Muscles

Hamstrings, glutes, quadriceps, gastrocnemus, peroneals, external rotators

Watchpoints

- Ensure the tips of the toes are the first to reach the ground after the jump, followed by the sole of the foot and then the heel. This order is reversed when rising from the ground.
- Keep the shoulders away from the ears
- Land softly and gracefully and allow the petit plié to break the impact
- Keep an upright, neutral spine

Contra-Indications

There is much more stress on the knee joint during this exercise as only one knee is taking the impact and therefore it is best avoided if there are any knee or ankle joint problems.

Standing side leg abduction

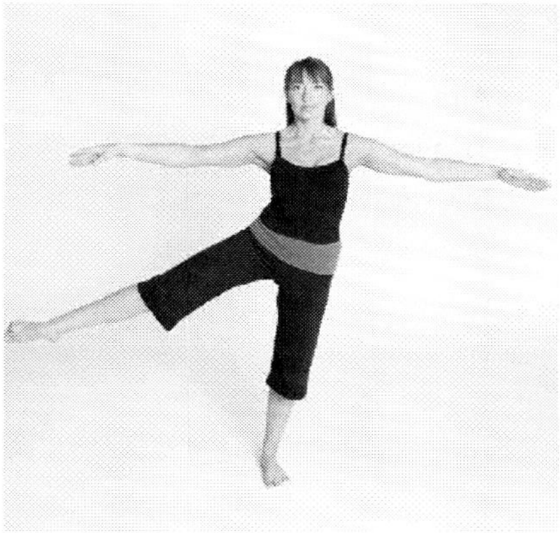

Aim

To strengthen the outer thighs, whilst maintaining a neutral spine and good posture

Starting Position

Stand upright with the feet in parallel and the legs adducted together and the arms in bras bas.

Action

Inhale - to prepare

Exhale - to engage the core abdominals and lift the leg out to the side whilst maintaining an upright posture. The leg is in a parallel position or may be slightly medially rotated and the arms open out to Second Position

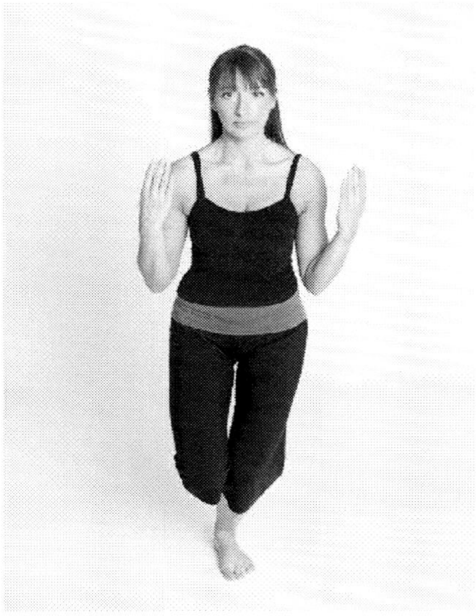

Inhale - to lower the leg and bend both knees into a demi plié in parallel. The working leg does not fully touch the floor

Exhale - to engage the core abdominals and raise the leg out once again. Repeat with the opposite leg

Hold the final leg abduction for a count of ten.

Target muscles

Glutes, quadriceps,

Watchpoints

- Ensure that the body does not lean forwards, backwards or sideways. Use the core abdominals to maintain good posture
- Try to keep both sides of the waist long and even to avoid hip hiking
- Ensure that both hip bones remain level to avoid any pelvic rotation
- Keep the distance between the ears and shoulders
- Maintain a neutral spine throughout
- Do not lock the knee joint

Contra-Indications

These exercises may place extra strain on the supporting knee joint so avoid if there is any discomfort for those with knee problems.

Standing back leg raises

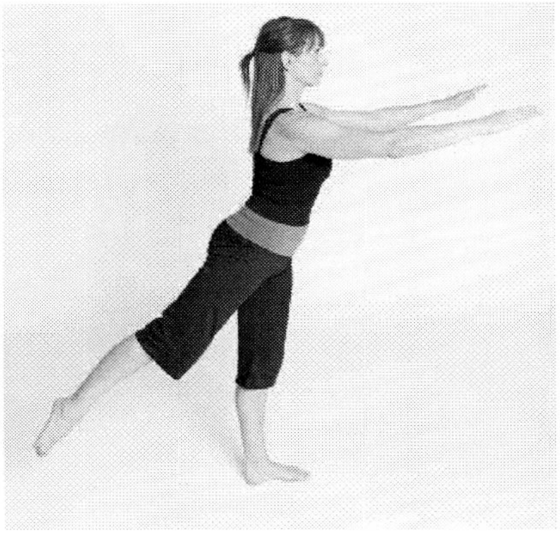

Aim

To strengthen the glutes, whilst maintaining a neutral spine and good posture

Starting Position

Stand upright with the feet in parallel and the legs adducted together and the arms in bras bas.

Action

Inhale - to prepare

Exhale - to engage the core abdominals and raise the leg back out behind the body whilst maintaining an upright posture. The leg is in a parallel position and the arms raise to First Position

Inhale - to lower the leg and bend both knees into a demi plié in parallel. The working leg does not fully touch the floor

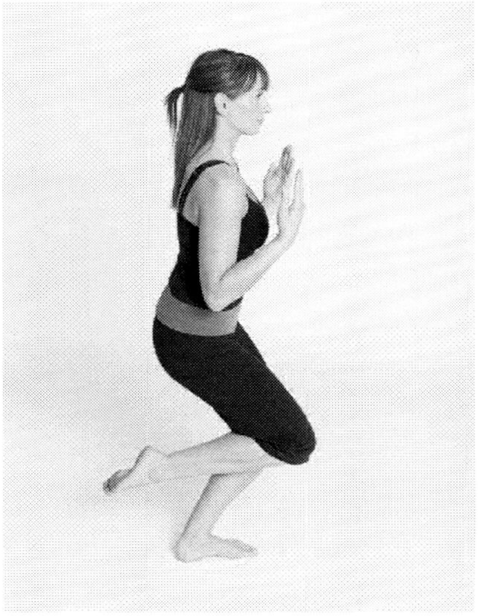

Exhale - to engage the core abdominals and raise the leg behind once again. Repeat with the opposite leg

Hold the final leg raise for a count of ten.

Target muscles

Glutes, quadriceps, hamstrings

Watchpoints

- Ensure that the body does not lean forwards, backwards or sideways. Use the core abdominals to maintain good posture
- Try to keep both sides of the waist long and even to avoid hip hiking
- Ensure that both hip bones remain level to avoid any pelvic rotation
- Keep the distance between the ears and shoulders
- Maintain a neutral spine throughout
- Do not lock the knee joint

Variation One (Adaptation)

Maintaining an upright posture whilst lifting the back leg up behind the body may cause some discomfort in the lower back. In this case, as the back leg raises behind, the body may lean forwards

Contra-Indications

These exercises may place extra strain on the supporting knee joint so avoid if there is any discomfort for those with knee problems. Chose variation one instead.

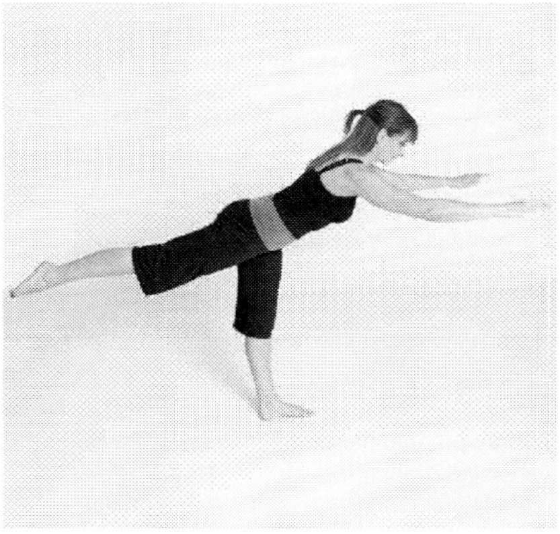

Variation One

Standing front leg raise

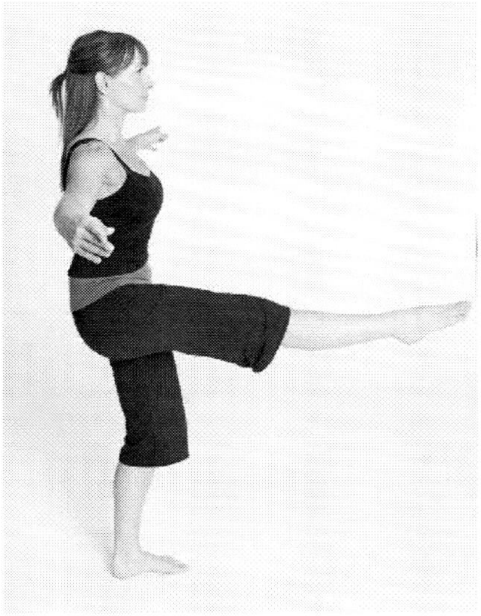

Aim

To strengthen the quadriceps, whilst maintaining a neutral spine and good posture

Starting Position

Stand upright with the feet in parallel and the legs adducted together and the arms in bras bas.

Action

Inhale - to prepare

Exhale - to engage the core abdominals and raise the leg up directly in front of the body, whilst maintaining an upright posture. The leg is in a parallel position and the arms open out to Second Position

Inhale - to lower the leg and bend both knees into a demi plié in parallel. The working leg does not fully touch the floor

Exhale - to engage the core abdominals and raise the leg forwards once again. Repeat with the opposite leg

Hold the final leg raise for a count of ten.

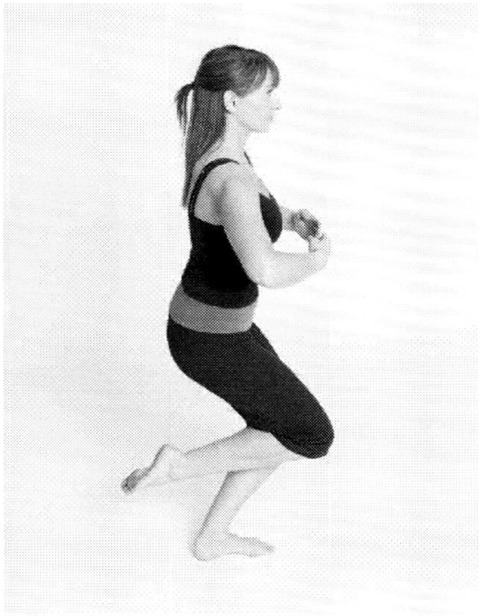

Target muscles

Glutes, quadriceps,

Watchpoints

- Ensure that the body does not lean forwards, backwards or sideways. Use the core abdominals to maintain good posture
- Try to keep both sides of the waist long and even to avoid hip hiking
- Ensure that both hip bones remain level to avoid any pelvic rotation
- Keep the distance between the ears and shoulders
- Maintain a neutral spine throughout
- Do not lock the knee joint

Contra-Indications

These exercises may place extra strain on the supporting knee joint so avoid if there is any discomfort for those with knee problems.

FLOORWORK

Leg and Butt Work
Quadricep Lean Backs with pelvic rocks
Thigh Press with pelvic rocks
The Table
Table with straight leg
Table with bent leg
Table with hamstring extension
Table with butt rotation
Awkward Plane
The Bullet
Side lying Developpé
Clam Shell
Leg Beats
Prone Frogs
Pelvic Lifts
The Hammock
The Bridge
Attitude in Mermaid
Torpedo
Cross Stitch

Upper Body Exercises
Press Up Preparation (Box Push ups)
Full Push Up
The Plank
Back leg pull
Plank Position – Lift opposite arm and leg
Side Plank
Oblique Plank
Reverse Plank
Dolphins
Tricep Press

Back Exercises
The Seesaw
Skydive
Mid back series
Cobra
The Eagle

Abdominal Work
Lean backs with chest press
Lean backs with arm release
Oblique Lean backs
Can Can
Oblique lean backs with knee lifts
Oblique curl ups
Criss Cross
Banana obliques
Pelvic Rocks
Reverse Curl
Toe Taps
Scissors
Diamond Leg Lowers
Double Leg Press
Double Leg Stretch
Floorwork Pliés
Frogs
Leg circles apart
Half curls up with leg abduction
Half curl up with leg raise
Full curl ups

Quadricep Lean Backs with Pelvic Rock

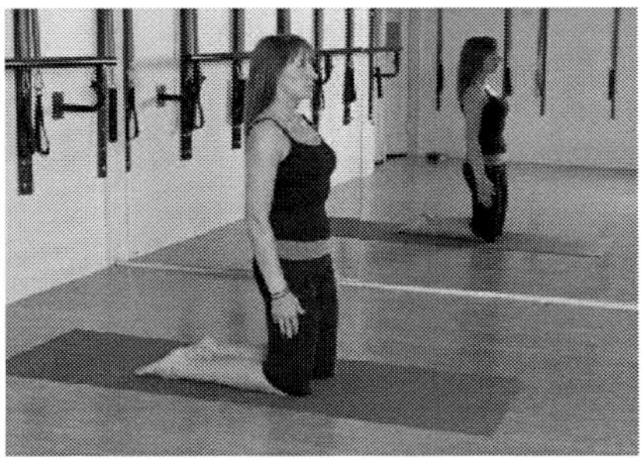

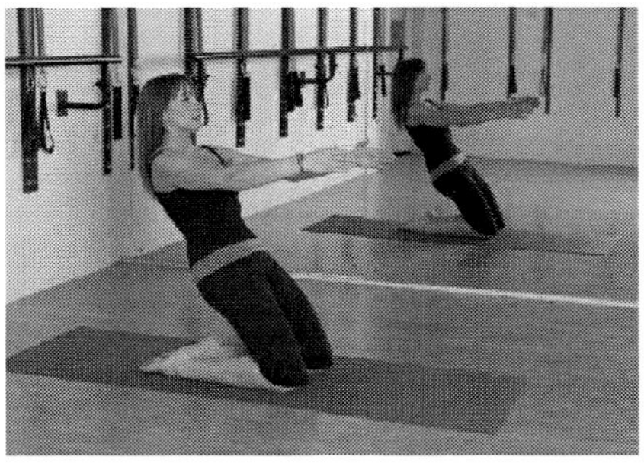

Aim

To work the quadriceps

Starting Position

Kneel upright with the knees and feet hip distance apart. The shoulders, hips and knees should be stacked on top of each other in a vertical alignment. The arms are in bras bas

Action

Inhale - to prepare

Exhale - engage the core abdominals and lean the body backwards from the knees (not the hips). The body should form a diagonal line from the knees, hips and shoulders. Simultaneously raise the arms to First position

Inhale – to prepare

Exhale – to engage the core abdominals and lean forwards to return the body to the starting position, bringing the arms back to bras bas. Repeat ten times.
Hold the lean back and perform twenty pelvic rocks, moving the pelvis quickly into a North position as lumber flexion increases and back to neutral again

Target Muscles

Quadriceps, core abdominals, gluteals

Watchpoints

- A neutral spine must be maintained at all times during the lean back
- Maintain distance between the ear and shoulder
- Keep the buttocks engaged to help prevent them from sticking out
- The movement comes from leaning backwards at the knee, not from the waist
- Only lean as far back as a neutral pelvis can be maintained
- Ensure that the back does not arch as the body leans backwards, particularly as the arm is raised up to shoulder height. Maintain good oblique engagement to prevent the ribs from flaring

Contra-Indications

This exercise places extra stress on the knee joints.

Thigh Press with Pelvic Rock

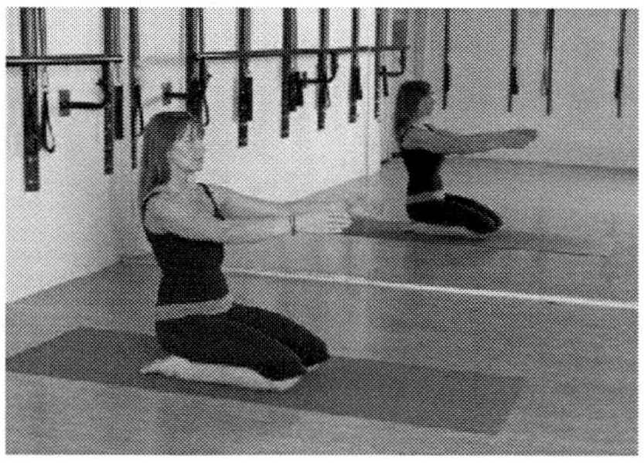

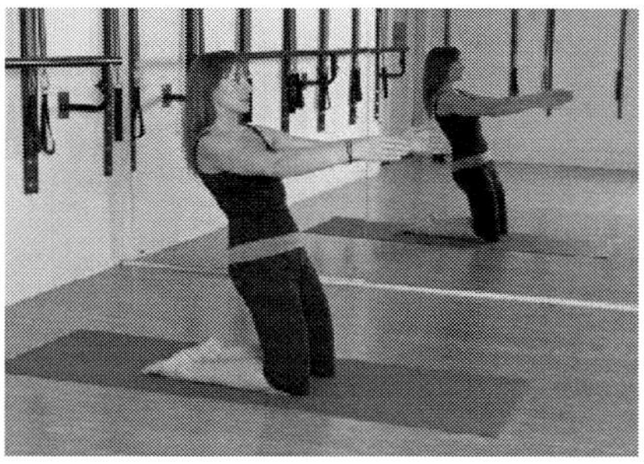

Aim

To work the quadriceps and gluteals

Starting Position

Kneel upright, sitting the buttocks on the heels. The shoulders, hips and knees should be stacked on top of each other in a vertical alignment. The arms are in bras bas

Action

Inhale - to prepare

Exhale - engage the core abdominals and the glutes to push the body forwards into an upright position. The body should form a straight line from the knees, hips and shoulders. Simultaneously raise the arms to First position

Inhale – to prepare

Exhale – to engage the core abdominals and return the body to the starting position, bringing the arms back to bras bas. Repeat ten times.

Hold the upright position on the final repetition and perform twenty pelvic rocks, moving the pelvis quickly into a North position as lumber flexion increases and back to neutral again

Target Muscles

Quadriceps, gluteals, core abdominals

Watchpoints

- A neutral spine must be maintained at all times during sitting and kneeling
- Maintain distance between the ear and shoulder
- Ensure the lumbar spine does not go into extension when pushing upright
- Ensure good core engagement to prevent the ribs from flaring

Contra-Indications

This exercise places extra stress on the knee joints and may be unsuitable for certain knee problems.

The Table

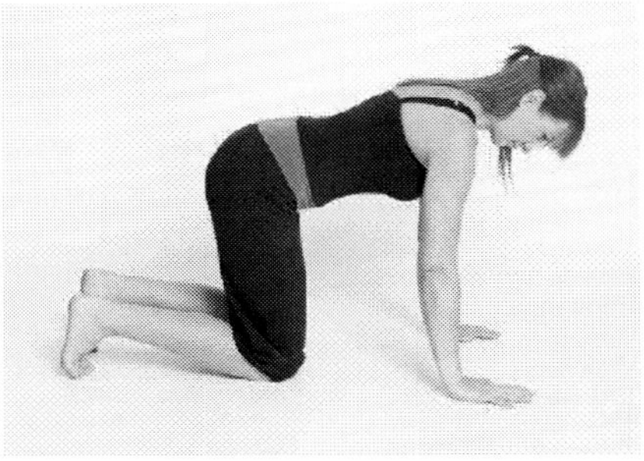

Aim

To work the core abdominals and quadriceps, whilst maintaining lumbar and scapula stability

Starting Position

Come to an all fours position with the knees bent directly under the hips and place the hands directly under the shoulders.

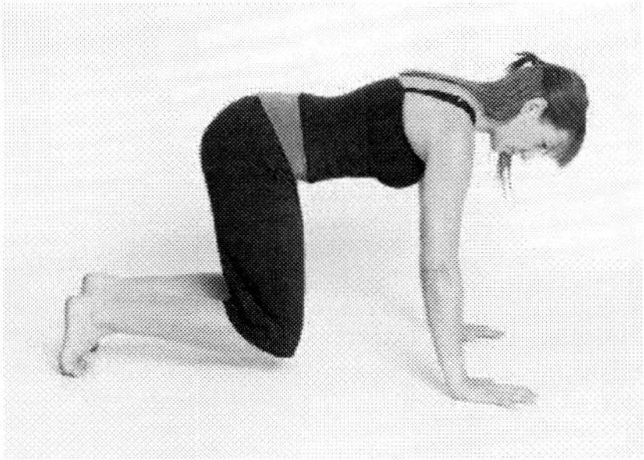

Action

Inhale - to prepare.

Exhale - to engage the core abdominals and raise the knees a few inches off the floor, maintaining a neutral spine. The closer the knees stay to the floor, the more challenging the position. Hold the position for up to ten seconds, breathing normally throughout. Lower the knees to the floor under control.

Target Muscles

Quadriceps, Core Abdominals

Watchpoints

- Try to lift both knees simultaneously to avoid lifting one ahead of the other
- Ensure a neutral spine is maintained when lifting and lowering the knees
- Try to avoid leaning forward as the knees lift off the floor as this reduces the workload for the legs and increases the workload for the upper body
- As the knees lift off the floor, try to keep the lumbar spine level with the shoulders to avoid sticking the buttocks in the air
- Ensure the shoulders stay away from the ear
- Try to avoid collapsing in between the shoulder blades. Engage serratus anterior to maintain the distance in between the shoulder blades

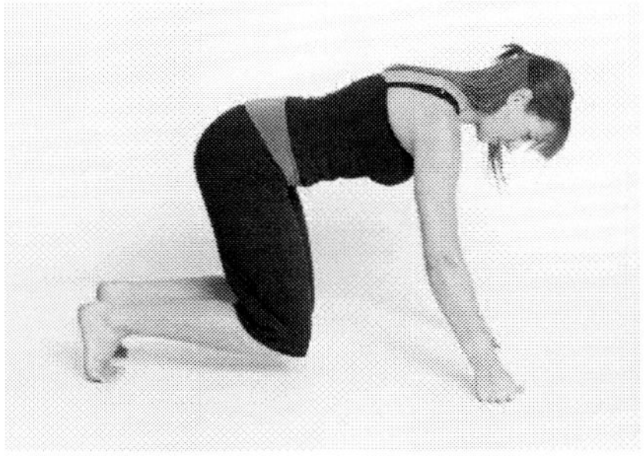

Variation One

Variation One (Adaptation)

To reduce pressure in the wrist joint, this exercise may be attempted on the knuckles of the hand, which will place the wrist in a more neutral position.

Variation Two (Progression)

To increase the workload for the legs, slightly lean back in the position so that the hips go behind the knees and the shoulders go behind the hands rather than being directly above them.

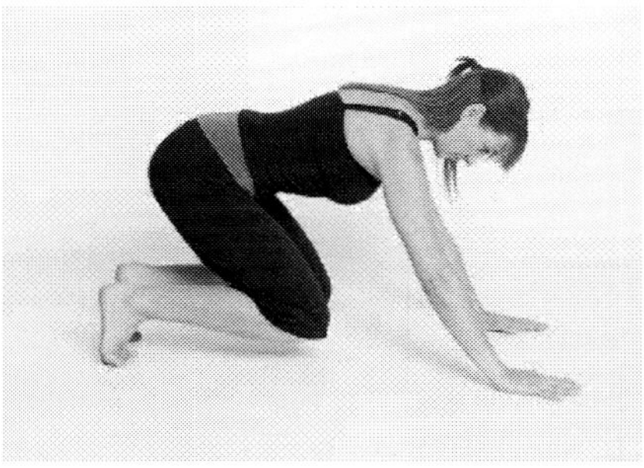

Variation One

Contra-Indications

This exercise places extra stress on the wrist and knee joints. Take extra care when attempting this exercise for certain clients with problems in these joints, as it may prove unsuitable for them.

Table with straight leg

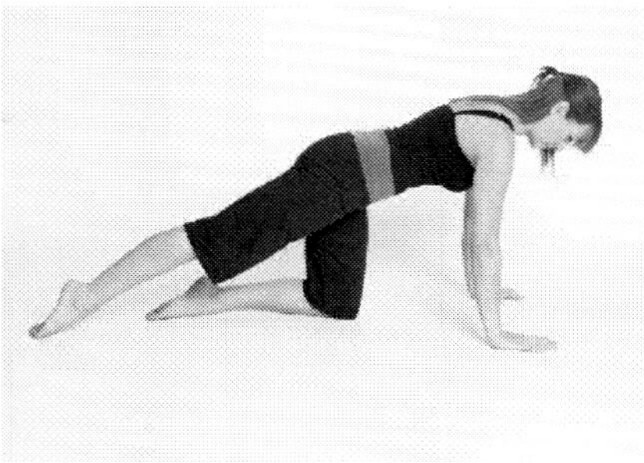

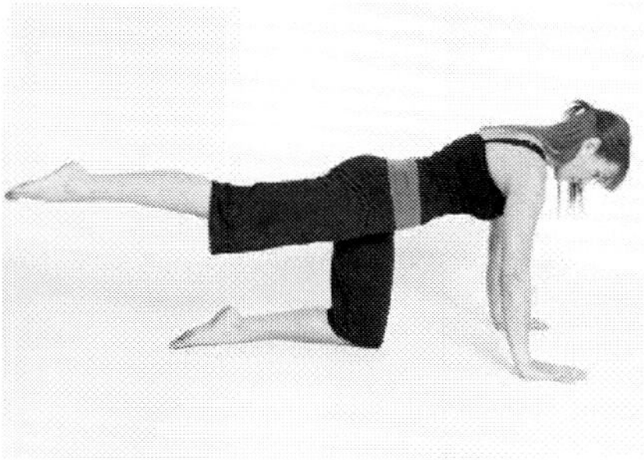

Aim

To work the glutes and core abdominals, whilst maintaining lumbar and scapula stability

Starting Position

Come to an all fours position with the knees bent directly under the hips and place the hands on the floor directly under the shoulders. Engage the core abdominals and fully straighten one leg along the floor and then lift the leg up in the air as high as a neutral pelvis can be maintained. Ideally the foot will be level with the spine and no higher

Action

Inhale - to prepare

Exhale - to engage the core abdominals raise the leg up an inch or two

Inhale – to lower the leg an inch or two, maintaining pelvic and scapula stability. Repeat with the opposite leg.

Target Muscles

Core Abdominals, glutes, scapula stabilisers

Watchpoints

- Ensure a neutral spine is maintained when lifting and lowering the leg
- Ensure the shoulders stay away from the ear
- Try to avoid collapsing in between the shoulder blades. Engage serratus anterior muscle to maintain the distance in between the shoulder blades
- Keep the waist long and even on both sides
- Keep the elbows soft

Variation One (Adaptation)

To reduce pressure in the wrist joint, this exercise may be attempted on the knuckles of the hand, which will place the wrist in a more neutral position (or on the elbows).

Variation Two (Adaptation)

This exercise may be performed lying face down on the floor for those with certain knee problems

Variation Three (Progression)

This exercise may be performed with both knees off the floor as for The Table exercise. This would be an extremely challenging exercise

Contra-Indications

This exercise places extra stress on the wrist and knee joints. Take extra care when attempting this exercise for certain clients with problems in these joints, as it may prove unsuitable for them. Choose variation one or two in this case.

Table with bent leg

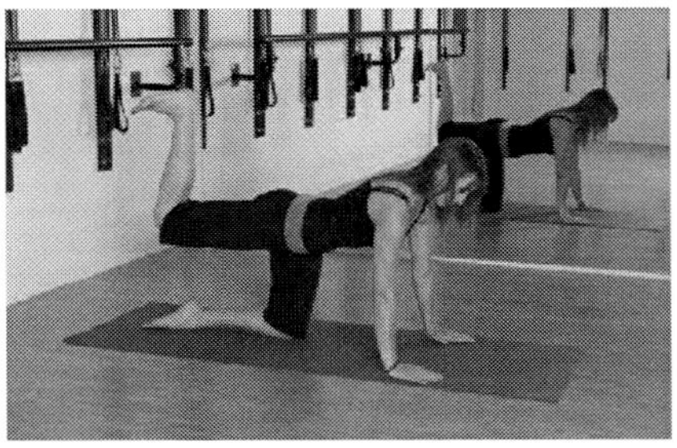

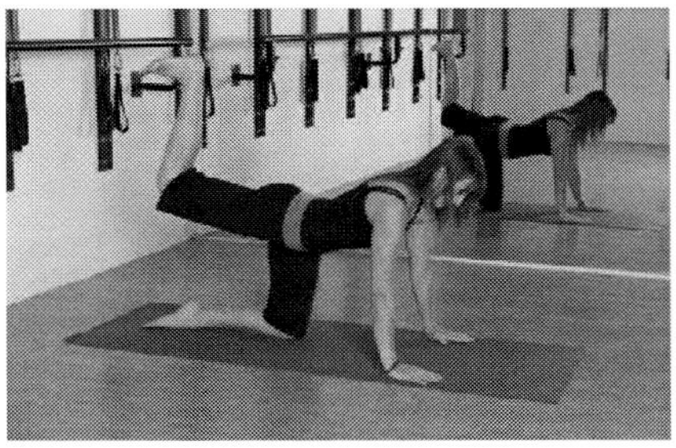

Aim

To work the glutes and core abdominals, whilst maintaining lumbar and scapula stability

Starting Position

Come to an all fours position with the knees bent directly under the hips and place the hands on the floor directly under the shoulders. Exhale to engage the core abdominals and stretch the right leg along the floor until it is fully straight and then lift it up in the air until it is level with the spine or as high as a neutral pelvis allows. Bend the knee at a 90 degree angle so that the foot is flexed and the sole of the foot faces the ceiling.

Action

Inhale - to prepare

Exhale - to engage the core abdominals and squeeze the glutes, pushing the sole of the foot upwards a few inches towards the ceiling, maintaining a 90 degree angle at the knee. Inhale to lower back down until the knee is once again level with the hip.

Inhale - to lower the leg back down again until the heel is level with the buttocks. Repeat with the opposite leg.

Target Muscles

Core Abdominals, hamstrings, glutes, scapula stabilisers

Watchpoints

- Ensure a neutral spine is maintained throughout the movement.
- Ensure the shoulders stay away from the ear. Try to avoid collapsing in between the shoulder blades. Engage serratus anterior muscle to maintain the distance in between the shoulder blades and keep the elbows soft.
- Keep the waist long and even on both sides and ensure that the knee does not go below the level of the hip

Variation One (Adaptation)

To reduce pressure in the wrist joint, this exercise may be attempted on the knuckles of the hand, which will place the wrist in a more neutral position (or on the elbows).

Variation Two (Adaptation)

This exercise may be performed lying face down on the floor for those with certain knee problems

Contra-Indications

This exercise places extra stress on the wrist and knee joints and may prove unsuitable for people with problems in these joints. Choose variation one or two in this case.

Table with hamstring extension

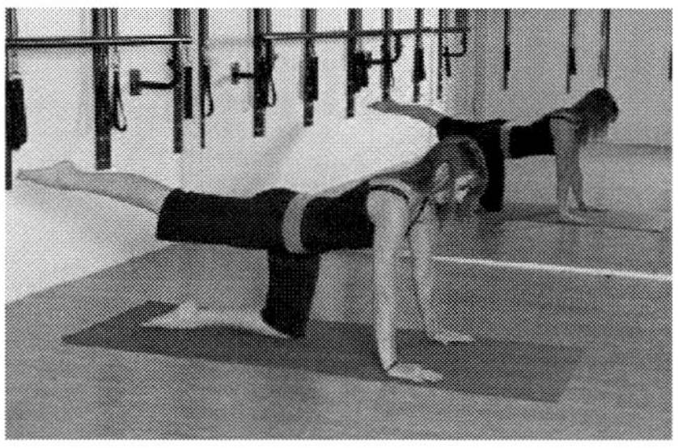

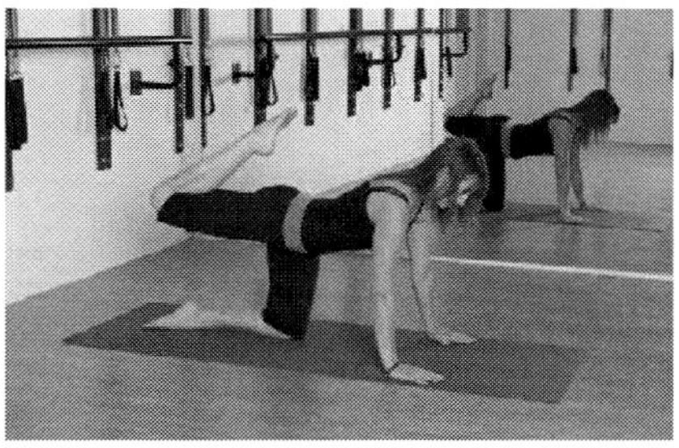

Aim

To work the glutes and core abdominals, whilst maintaining lumbar and scapula stability

Starting Position

Come to an all fours position with the knees bent directly under the hips and place the hands on the floor directly under the shoulders. Exhale to engage the core abdominals and stretch the right leg along the floor until it is fully straight and then lift it up in the air until it is level with the spine or as high as a neutral pelvis allows.

Action

Inhale - to prepare

Exhale - to engage the core abdominals and bend the knee so that the heel comes towards the buttocks

Inhale - to straighten the leg back out again until the heel is level with the buttocks. Bend and straighten the leg for up to 10 repetitions. Repeat with the opposite leg.

Target Muscles

Core Abdominals, hamstrings, glutes, scapula stabilisers

Watchpoints

- When the knee bends ensure that the knee does not lose height. Ideally the ankle, knee and hip will be level when the leg is straight. As the knee bends, it stays level with the hip, whilst the heel moves towards the bottom.
- Ensure a neutral spine is maintained when bending and straightening the leg
- Ensure the shoulders stay away from the ear. Try to avoid collapsing in between the shoulder blades. Engage serratus anterior muscle to maintain the distance in between the shoulder blades and keep the elbows soft.
- Keep the waist long and even on both sides and both ASIS level

Variation One (Adaptation)

To reduce pressure in the wrist joint, this exercise may be attempted on the knuckles of the hand, which will place the wrist in a more neutral position (or on the elbows).

Variation Two (Adaptation)

This exercise may be performed lying face down on the floor for those with certain knee problems

Contra-Indications

This exercise places extra stress on the wrist and knee joints and may prove unsuitable for people with problems in these joints. Choose variation one or two in this case.

Table with butt rotation

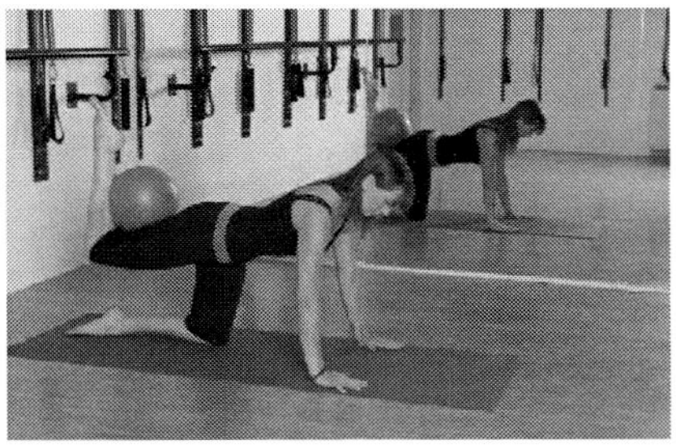

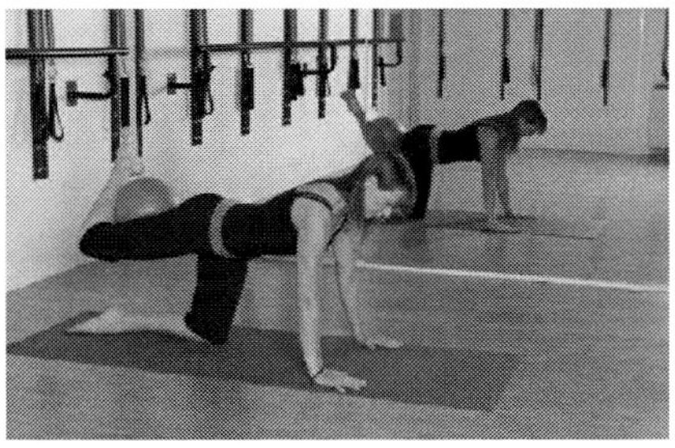

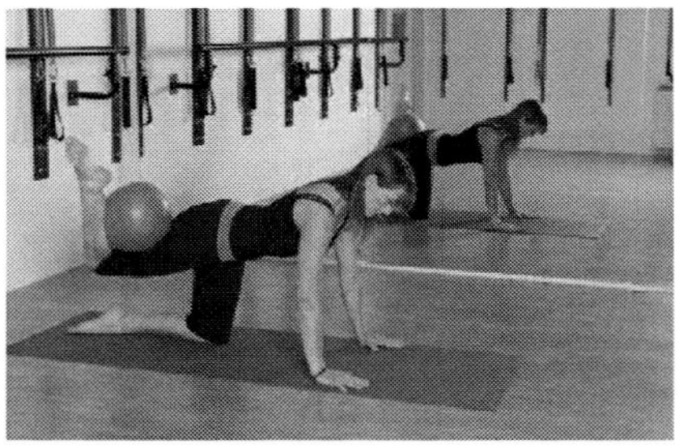

Aim

To work the glutes and core abdominals, whilst maintaining lumbar and scapula stability

Starting Position

Come to an all fours position with the knees bent directly under the hips and place the hands on the floor directly under the shoulders. Exhale to engage the core abdominals and stretch the right leg along the floor until it is fully straight and then lift it up in the air until it is level with the spine or as high as a neutral pelvis allows. Bend the knee to a 90 degree angle. A ball may be used as illustrated.

Action

Inhale - to prepare

Exhale - to engage the core abdominals and externally rotate the leg out in the hip socket, whilst maintaining the 90 degree angle

Inhale - to rotate the leg back into parallel

Exhale - to engage the core abdominals and internally rotate the leg out in the hip socket, whilst maintaining the 90 degree angle

Repeat with the opposite leg.

Target Muscles

Core Abdominals, hamstrings, glutes, scapula stabilisers

Watchpoints

- As the leg rotates, ensure that it stays at the same height
- Ensure a neutral spine is maintained when moving the leg
- Ensure the shoulders stay away from the ear. Try to avoid collapsing in between the shoulder blades. Engage serratus anterior muscle to maintain the distance in between the shoulder blades and keep the elbows soft.
- Keep the waist long and even on both sides and both ASIS level

Variation One (Adaptation)

To reduce pressure in the wrist joint, this exercise may be attempted on the knuckles of the hand, which will place the wrist in a more neutral position (or on the elbows).

Variation Two (Adaptation)

This exercise may be performed lying face down on the floor for those with certain knee problems

Variation Three (Progression)

This exercise may be performed as above but with the knee straight and the leg extended out at 90 degrees

Contra-Indications

This exercise places extra stress on the wrist and knee joints and may prove unsuitable for people with problems in these joints. Choose variation one or two in this case. A turned out position of the leg may be unsuitable for sciatica.

Awkward Plane

Aim

To work the abductors, adductors and core abdominals, whilst maintaining lumbar and scapula stability

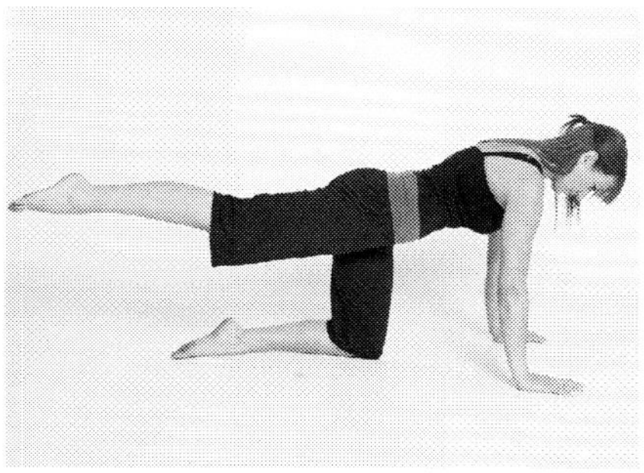

Starting Position

Come to an all fours position with the knees bent directly under the hips and place the hands on the floor directly under the shoulders. Engage the core abdominals and fully straighten one leg along the floor and then lift the leg up in the air as high as a neutral pelvis can be maintained. Ideally the foot will be level with the spine and no higher

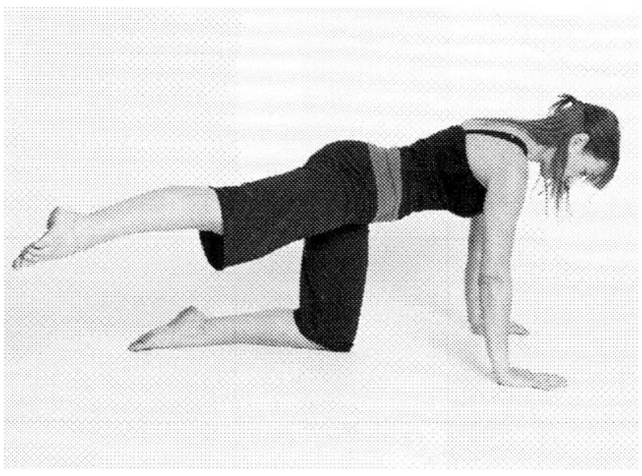

Action

Inhale - to prepare

Exhale - to engage the core abdominals and abduct the leg sideways, keeping an even height as the leg moves outwards

Inhale – to adduct the leg back into the midline again, maintaining pelvic and scapula stability.

Repeat with the opposite leg.

Target Muscles

Core Abdominals, glutes, scapula stabilisers, adductors

Watchpoints

- Ensure a neutral spine is maintained when lifting and lowering the leg
- Ensure the shoulders stay away from the ear
- Try to avoid collapsing in between the shoulder blades. Engage serratus anterior muscle to maintain the distance in between the shoulder blades
- Keep the waist long and even on both sides
- Ensure the shoulders stay level with each other
- Keep the elbows soft and ensure that one elbow does not bend more than the other
- Try to avoid leaning the body weight over to one side as the leg abducts
- Only move the leg as far as a neutral pelvis allows

Variation One (Adaptation)

To reduce pressure in the wrist joint, this exercise may be attempted on the knuckles of the hand, which will place the wrist in a more neutral position (or on the elbows).

Variation Two (Adaptation)

This exercise may be performed lying face down on the floor for those with certain knee problems

Contra-Indications

This exercise places extra stress on the wrist and knee joints. Take extra care when attempting this exercise for certain clients with problems in these joints, as it may prove unsuitable for them. Choose variation one or two in this case.

The Bullet

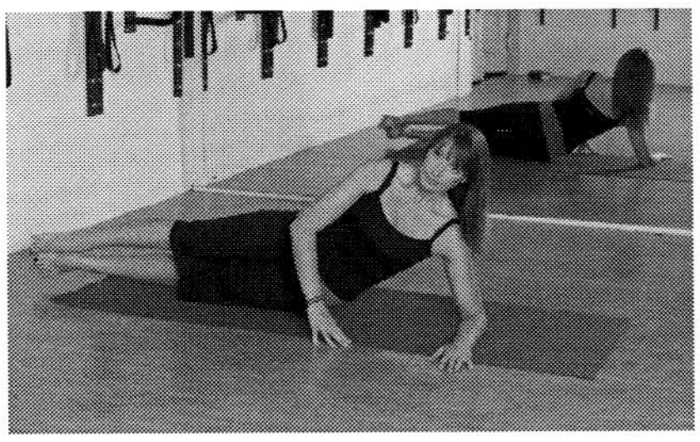

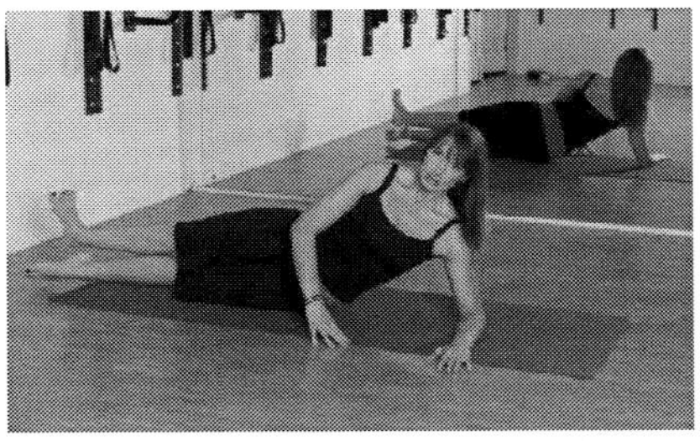

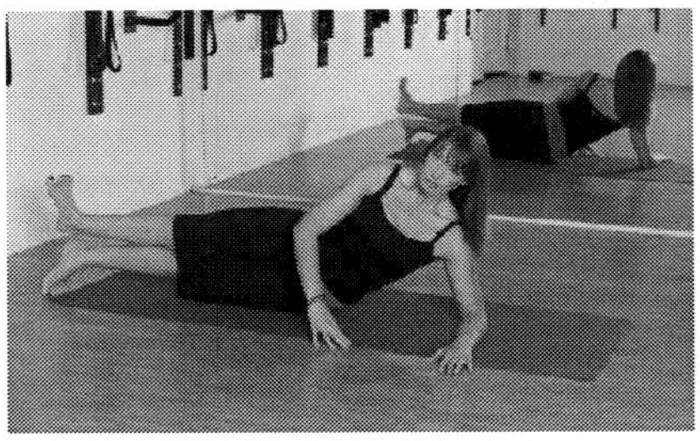

Variation One

Aim

To work the gluteals and external rotators, whilst maintaining length in the waist and good pelvic stability

Starting Position

Lie on left hand side of the body with the left arm outstretched above the head. A small head cushion may be placed between the ear and shoulder. The right hand is resting on the floor in front of the body. Both legs are straight with feet, knee and hips stacked joint over joint and in alignment with the spine. Alternatively, the body may be propped up on the supporting elbow (as illustrated)

Action

Inhale - To engage the core abdominals, lengthen the waist and raise both legs up off the floor

Exhale – To externally rotate the legs out in the hip socket

Inhale - To internally rotate the legs back to parallel again

Target Muscles

Gluteals, external rotators

Watchpoints

- Ensure the shoulders stay away from the ear and the gap between ear and shoulder remains equal on both sides
- Try to keep the length on both sides of the waist to avoid the tendency to shorten in the waist on the top side
- Keep the collar bones open
- Ensure that the hips are stacked joint over joint to avoid the tendency for the pelvis to roll back
- Ensure that the buttocks do not stick out or the knees bend as the legs externally rotate

Variation One (Adaptation)

This may be performed with the legs on the floor if discomfort is felt in the lower back.

Contra-Indications

External rotation may not be suitable for sciatica. Side lying exercises with both legs in the air can place extra strain on one side of the lower back. If discomfort is felt, then choose Variation One instead.

Side lying Developpé

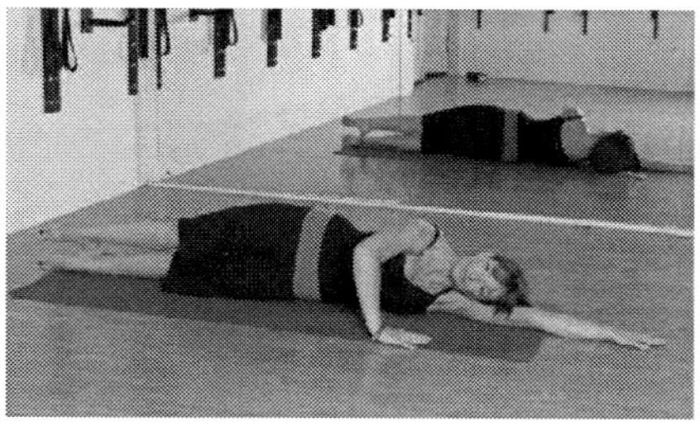

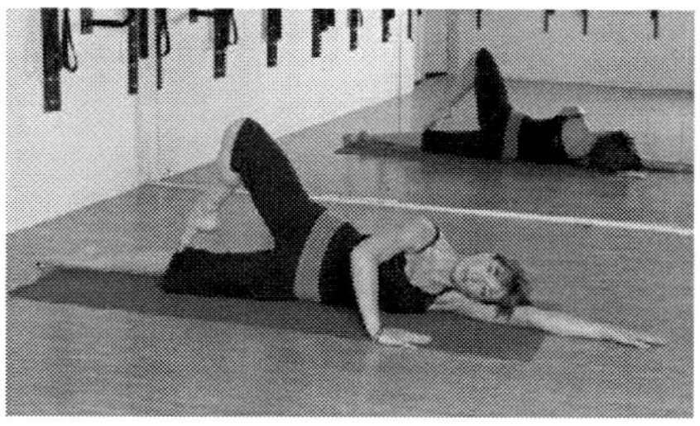

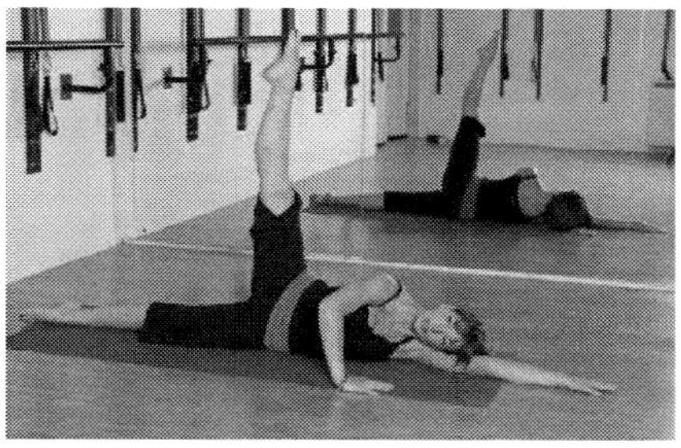

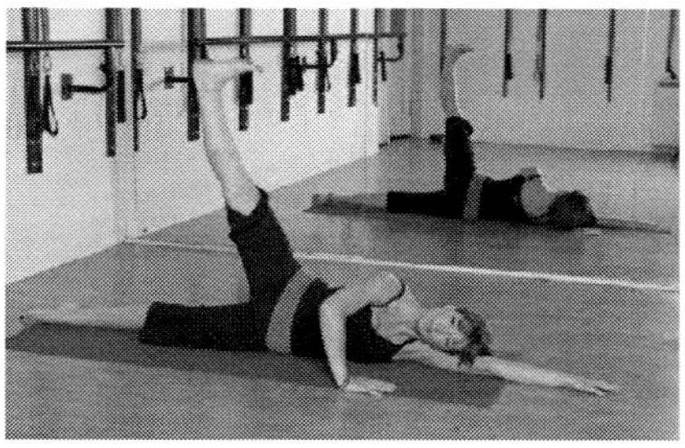

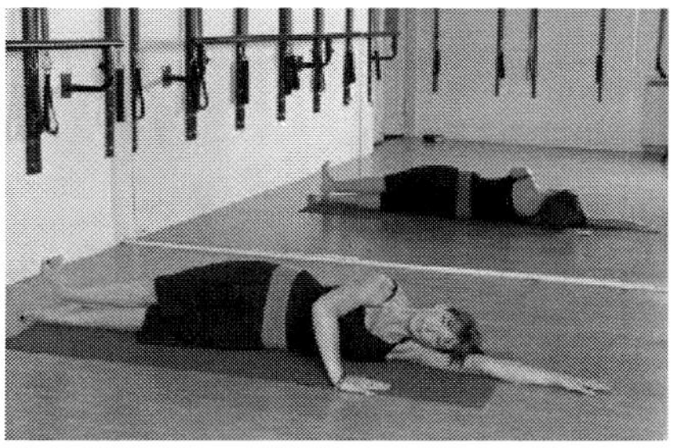

Aim

To work the abductors and adductors whilst maintaining length in the waist and good pelvic stability

Starting Position

Lie on left hand side of the body with the left arm outstretched above the head. The right hand is resting on the floor in front of the body. Both legs are straight with feet, knee and hips stacked joint over joint and in alignment with the spine.

Action

Exhale – Engage the core abdominals and externally rotate the top leg out in the hip socket. Simultaneously bend the knee of the top leg and draw the foot up along the inside of the bottom leg until the toes of the top leg reach the inside of the knee on the bottom leg

Inhale – To straighten the knee, extending the leg up towards the ceiling

Exhale – To flex the foot, engage the adductors and draw the top leg down slowly to meet the bottom leg, still in external rotation

Inhale – To point the toes and then repeat again

Target Muscles

Gluteals, external rotators, adductors, hip flexors, gastrocnemius, soleus

Watchpoints

- Ensure the shoulders stay away from the ear and the gap between ear and shoulder remains equal on both sides
- Try to keep the length on both sides of the waist to avoid the tendency to shorten in the waist on the top side
- Keep the collar bones open
- The work in this exercise comes from the use of opposition. Try to lengthen not only the waist but also the top leg. Push the top leg diagonally away to encourage more length.
- Ensure that the hips are stacked joint over joint to avoid the tendency for the pelvis to roll back if the leg is lifted too high

Variation One (Progression)

This may be performed with the bottom leg off the floor for added challenge

Contra-Indications

External rotation may not be suitable for sciatica. Side lying exercises with both legs in the air can place extra strain on one side of the lower back. If discomfort is felt, then choose Variation One instead.

Clam Shell

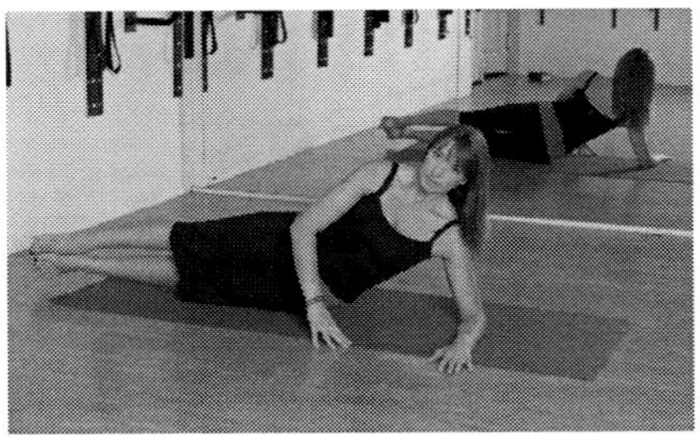

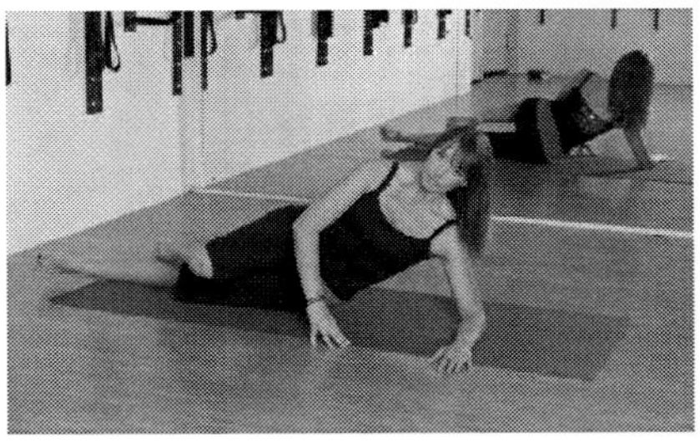

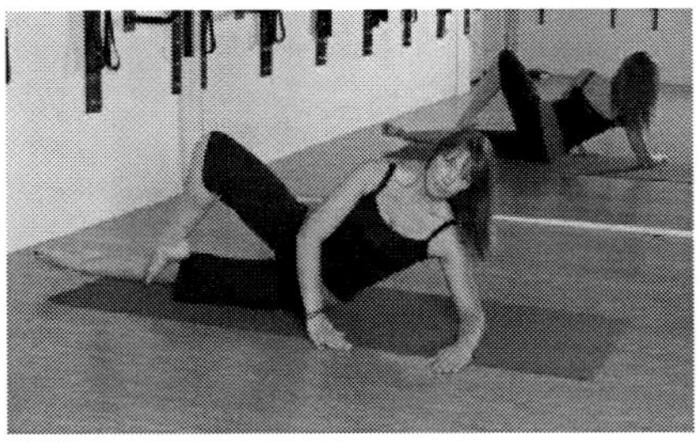

Aim

To work the gluteals, whilst maintaining length in the waist and good pelvic stability

Starting Position

Lie on left hand side of the body with the left arm outstretched above the head. The right hand is resting on the floor in front of the body. Both legs are straight with feet, knee and hips stacked joint over joint and in alignment with the spine. Alternatively, the body may be propped up on the supporting elbow (as illustrated). Engage the core abdominals and raise both legs up off the floor. Bend the knee of the top leg and draw the foot up along the inside of the bottom leg until the toes of the top leg reach the inside of the knee on the bottom leg.

Action

Exhale – To externally rotate the top thigh outwards so that the knee is pointing up to the ceiling as far as a stable pelvis allows. Simultaneously externally rotate the bottom leg out in the hip socket

Inhale – To internally rotate both legs back into parallel, lowering the top knee back to the start position

Target Muscles

Gluteals, external rotators

Watchpoints

- Ensure the shoulders stay away from the ear and the gap between ear and shoulder remains equal on both sides
- Try to keep the length on both sides of the waist to avoid the tendency to shorten in the waist on the top side
- Keep the collar bones open
- The work in this exercise comes from the use of opposition. Try to lengthen not only the waist but also the top knee. Push the top knee diagonally away to encourage more length.
- Ensure that the hips are stacked joint over joint to avoid the tendency for the pelvis to roll back if the knee is lifted too high

Variation One (Adaptation)

This may be performed with the bottom leg on the floor if discomfort is felt in the lower back.

Variation Two (Progression)

Add an internal rotation. After the initial external rotation, keep the knees together but lift the top foot upwards. Alternate lifting the knee and then foot (i.e. one internal rotation with one external rotation).

Contra-Indications

External rotation may not be suitable for sciatica. Side lying exercises with both legs in the air can place extra strain on one side of the lower back. If discomfort is felt, then choose Variation One instead.

Leg Beats

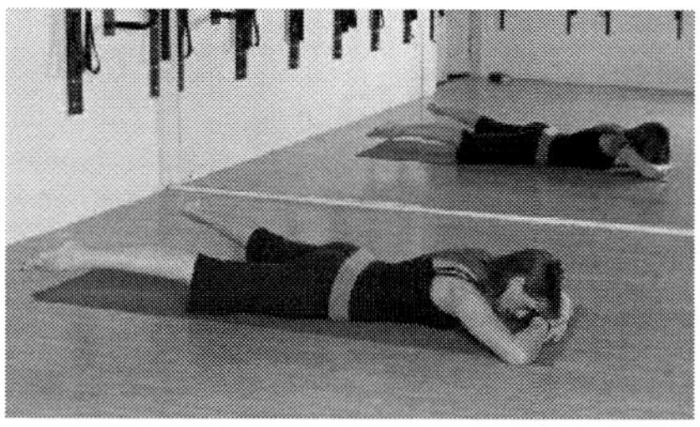

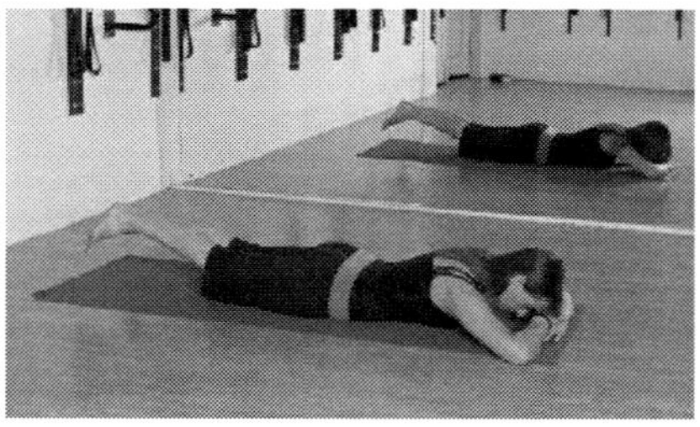

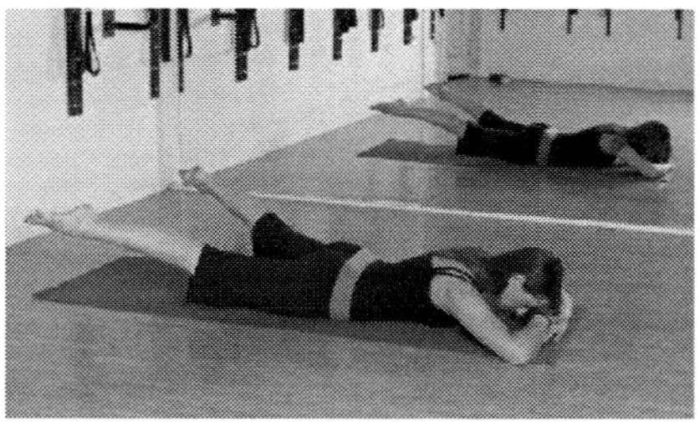

Aim

To work in turn out, whist strengthening the gluteals and to maintain scapula stability

Starting Position

Lie prone with legs adducted and externally rotated in the hip sockets. The feet are flexed. Bend the elbows and rest the forehead on the back of the hands.

Action

Inhale - to prepare and raise both legs off the floor a few inches

Exhale - engage the powerhouse and open out the legs to the sides a few inches, maintaining the height of the legs

Inhale - to close the legs together again

Target Muscles

Core abdominals, gluteals, adductors, scapula stabilisers, erector spinae, quadriceps

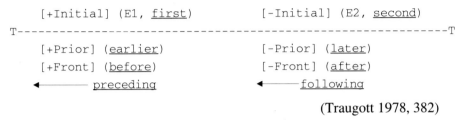

Watchpoints

- Ensure the core abdominals are engaged throughout
- Maintain the length between the ears and shoulders and try to avoid collapsing in between the shoulder blades or shortening at the back of the neck
- Maintain the length between the ears and shoulders and try to avoid collapsing in between the shoulder blades. Engage serratus anterior muscle to maintain the distance in between the shoulder blades
- Maintain connection in the inner thighs throughout (not just when closing the legs)
- Try to maintain engagement of the quadriceps to prevent the knees from bending
- Try to ensure that the heels touch when closing the legs

Variation One (Adaptation)

This exercise may be done in a parallel leg position

Variation Two (Adaptation)

This exercise may be done without the legs being raised in the air. Perform as above with both legs on the floor in either parallel or in turnout

Contra-Indications

This exercise may be unsuitable for sciatica because of the turned out position. Chose variation one instead. Raising both legs in the air may cause excessive strain on the lumbar spine and be uncomfortable for certain back problems or lordotic postures. A cushion may be placed under the hips to help alleviate this problem. If discomfort is still felt, then choose Variation Two.

Prone Frogs

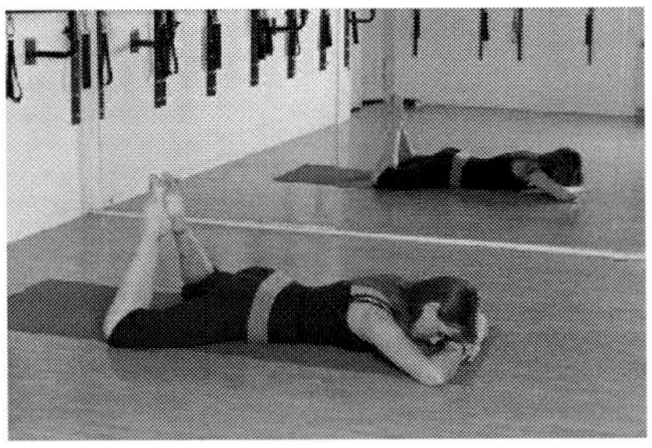

Aim

To work in turn out, whist strengthening the gluteals and to maintain scapula stability

Starting Position

Lie prone with the legs shoulder distance apart and externally rotated in the hip sockets. The feet are pointed. Bend the knees and bring the heels together, whilst keeping the knees apart. Alternatively, the feet may be flexed, so that the sole of the foot faces the ceiling and the knees are bent at 90 degrees. Bend the elbows and rest the forehead on the back of the palms.

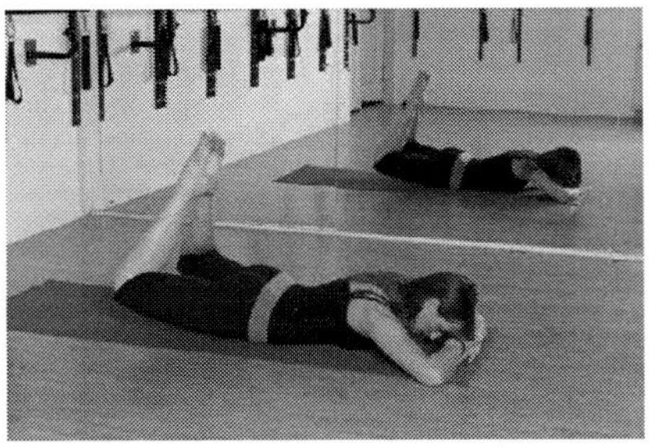

Action

Inhale - to prepare

Exhale – to raise both thighs off the floor a few inches, maintaining the angle at the knee

Inhale - to lower the legs to the floor again

Target Muscles

Core abdominals, gluteals, adductors, scapula stabilisers, erector spinae, quadriceps

Watchpoints

- Ensure the core abdominals are engaged throughout
- Maintain length at the back of the neck
- Maintain a 90 degree angle at the knee
- Maintain the length between the ears and shoulders and try to avoid collapsing in between the shoulder blades.

Variation One (Adaptation)

This exercise may be done in a parallel leg position

Variation Two (Adaptation)

This exercise may be done without both legs being in the air if this places discomfort on the lower back. Raise only one leg at a time, alternating between right and left.

Variation Three (Progression)

Once the legs have lifted up into a frog, straighten the knees, opening out the legs to the side, maintaining the height of the legs. Continue flexing and extending the knees, whilst maintaining the thighs off the floor

Contra-Indications

This exercise may be unsuitable for sciatica because of the turned out position. Chose variation one instead. Raising both legs in the air may cause excessive strain on the lumbar spine and be uncomfortable for certain back problems or lordotic postures. A cushion may be placed under the hips to help alleviate this problem or choose Variation Two. If discomfort is still felt, then this exercise is best avoided.

Pelvic Lifts

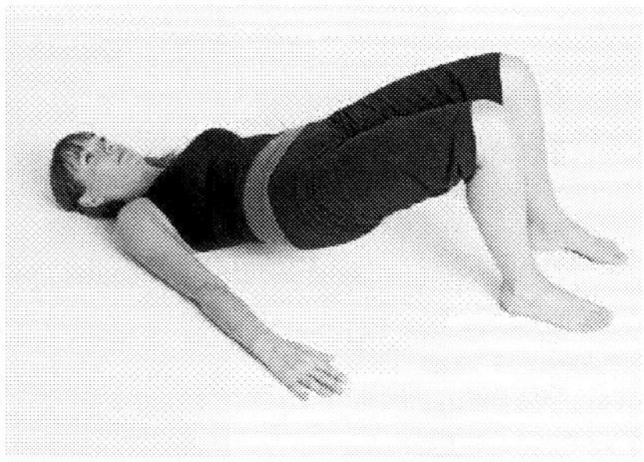

Aim

Starting Position

Lie supine on the floor in the relaxation position. Engage the core abdominals and tilt the pelvis into a posterior tilt and gently peel the spine off the floor, one vertebra at a time until a neutral bridge position is achieved (i.e. knee, hip and shoulder form a diagonal straight line with the lumbar spine in neutral). The arms are down by the sides of the body on the floor.

Action

Inhale - to prepare.

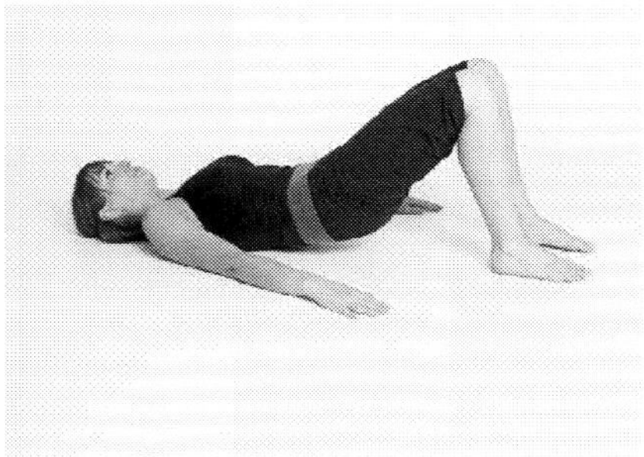

Exhale - to engage the core abdominals and squeeze the buttocks tightly and rock the pelvis into a posterior tilt. The pelvis may lift an inch or two but ensure that the lumbar spine does not go into extension

Inhale - to lower the pelvis back down a few inches and return to neutral, maintaining gluteal engagement. Repeat up to twenty times.

Exhale - to lower the torso back down to the floor, one vertebra at a time when finished

Target muscles

Core abdominals, hamstrings, gluteals

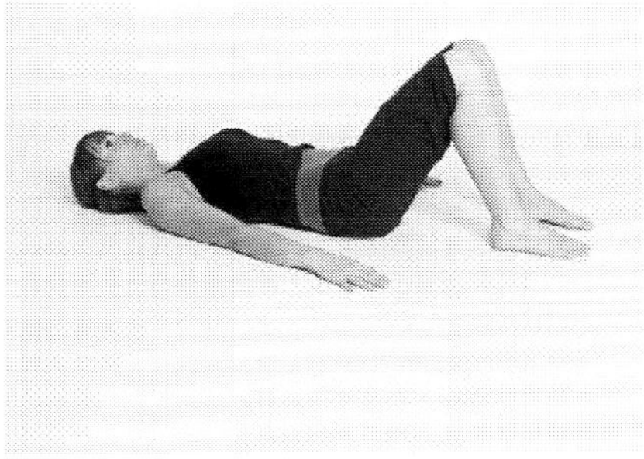

Watchpoints

- Ensure the shoulders stay away from the ears
- Watch the back does not arch. Only lift the pelvis as much as a stable spine can be maintained
- Try to ensure the lift comes from engaging the gluteal muscles to push the pelvis up and not by lifting the spine higher

Variation One (Progression)

Lift the arms off the floor for extra challenge and added balance work

Variation Two (Progression)

Perform the exercise with one leg in the air, bent at 90 degrees above the hips and squeeze the buttocks of the working leg on the floor.

Contra-Indications

Avoid "bridging" (i.e. arching the back by lifting the spine too high), as this will place stress on the lower back. In some cases, even a neutral position of the lumbar spine can cause discomfort. In these cases, the exercise may be performed with a posterior pelvic tilt rather than in a neutral position. More of the thoracic spine will be in contact with the floor in this instance and therefore the body in general will be lower and closer to the floor.

The Hammock

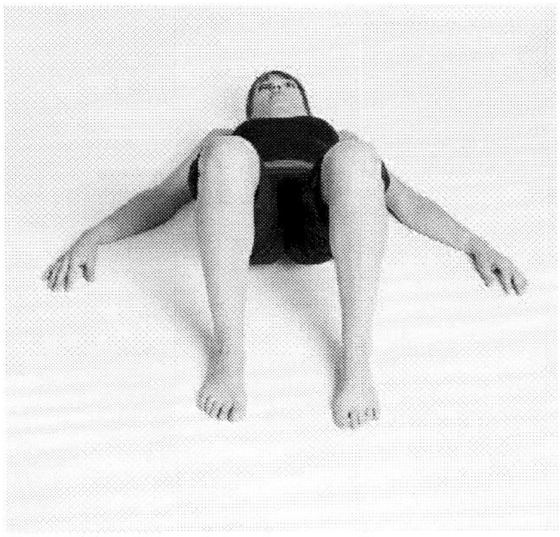

Aim

Starting Position

Lie supine on the floor in the relaxation position. Engage the core abdominals and tilt the pelvis into a posterior tilt and gently peel the lumbar spine off the floor. The arms are down by the sides of the body on the floor.

Action

Inhale - to engage the core abdominals and gently sway the pelvis a few inches to the left so that the hips are to the left of the knees and therefore out of alignment.

Exhale – to squeeze the left buttock and raise the pelvis up a few inches

Inhale - to lower the pelvis back down a few inches and return to the centre, maintaining gluteal engagement

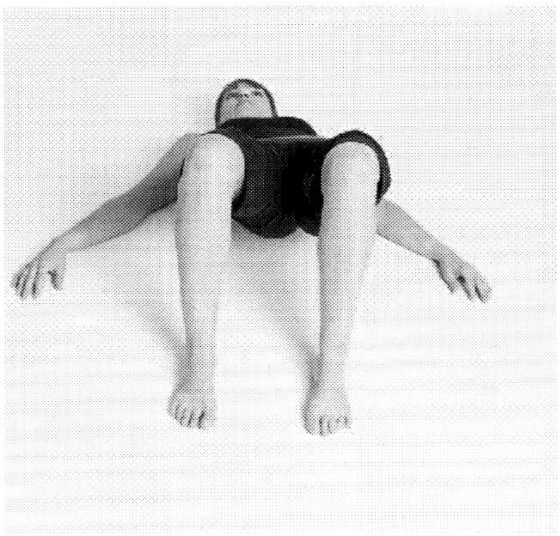

Inhale - to engage the core abdominals and gently sway the pelvis a few inches to the right so that the hips are to the right of the knees and therefore out of alignment.

Exhale – to squeeze the right buttock and raise the pelvis up a few inches

Inhale - to lower the pelvis back down a few inches and return to the centre, maintaining gluteal engagement.

Exhale - to lower the torso back down to the floor, one vertebra at a time when finished

Target muscles

Core abdominals, hamstrings, gluteals

Watchpoints

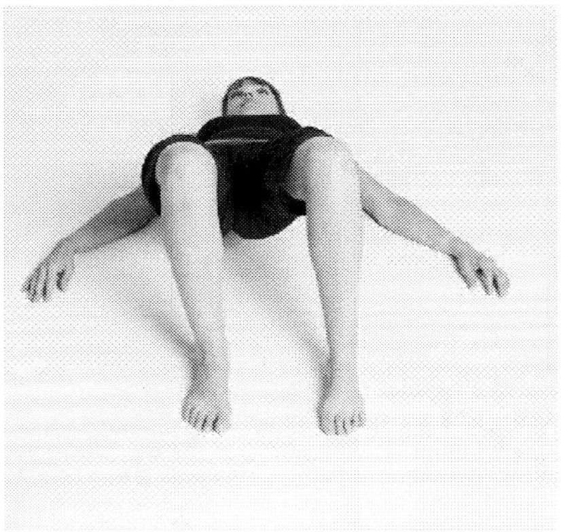

- Ensure the shoulders stay away from the ears
- Ensure the lumbar spine does not go into extension. Only lift the pelvis as much as a stable spine can be maintained
- Try to ensure the lift comes from engaging the gluteal muscles to push the pelvis up and not by lifting the spine higher

Variation One (Progression)

Lift the arms off the floor for extra challenge and added balance work

Variation Two (Progression)

Perform the exercise with one leg in the air, bent at 90 degrees above the hips and squeeze the buttocks of the working leg on the floor.

Contra-Indications

Avoid "bridging" (i.e. arching the back by lifting the spine too high), as this will place stress on the lower back. In some cases, even a neutral position of the lumbar spine can cause discomfort. In these cases, the exercise may be performed with a posterior pelvic tilt rather than in a neutral position. More of the thoracic spine will be in contact with the floor in this instance and therefore the body in general will be lower and closer to the floor.

The Bridge

Aim

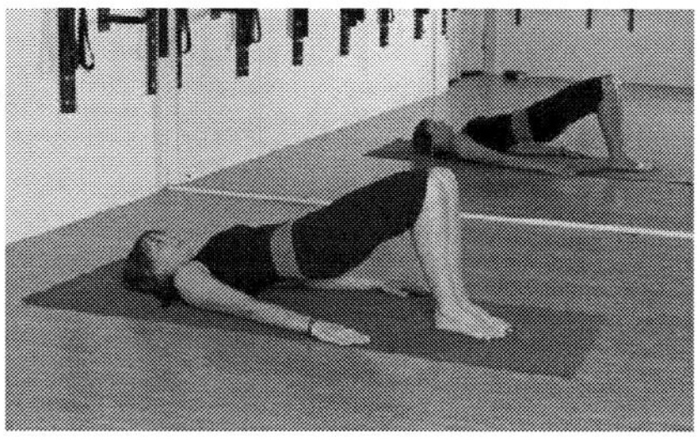

To maintain a strong bridge position with neutral pelvis and also maintain an equal height in the pelvis. The hip bones should be level with each other.

Starting Position

Lie supine on the floor in the relaxation position with knees bent and the legs adducted together. Inhale to prepare. Exhale to engage the core abdominals and tilt the pelvis into a posterior tilt and gently peel the spine off the floor, one vertebra at a time until a neutral bridge position is achieved (i.e. knee, hip and shoulder form a diagonal straight line with the lumbar spine in neutral).

Action

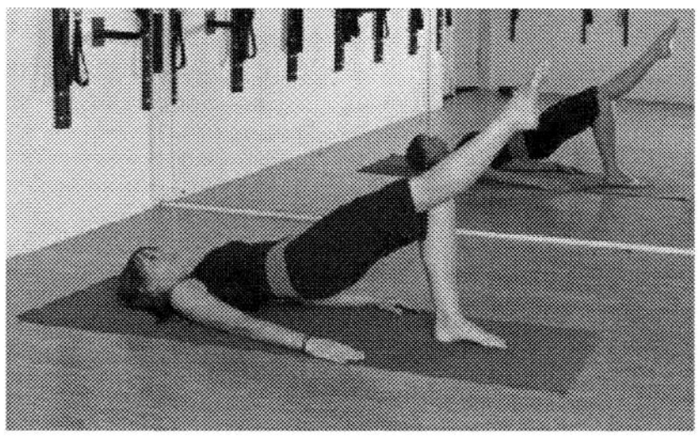

Exhale - To engage the core abdominals and extend the right knee directly in front until the foot is off the floor with the leg fully straight. The legs remain adducted and the knees are glued together and the ASIS level. Hold for up to ten counts breathing normally throughout

Inhale - To flex the knee and return the foot back down to the floor gently. Repeat with the opposite leg.

Repeat the above sequence but raise the heels off the floor and bring the feet to demi pointe. Repeat with the opposite leg.

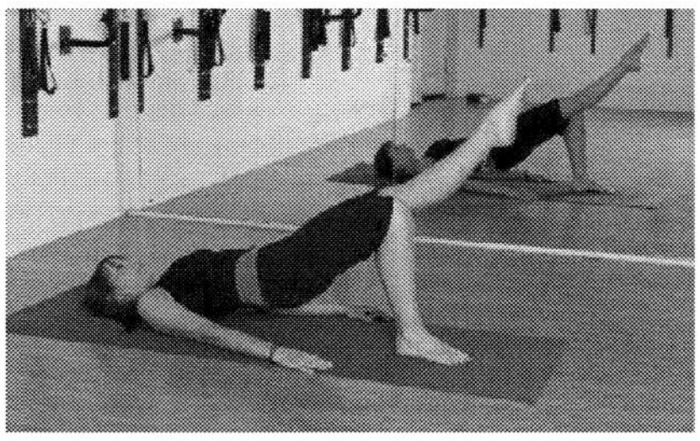

Repeat the above sequence but flex the feet and raise the toes off the floor so that only the heels remain in contact with the floor. Repeat with the opposite leg.

Target Muscles

Core abdominals, hamstrings, gluteals, quadriceps, gastrocnemus, soleus

Watchpoints

- Use the glutes to keep the pelvis at a constant height to avoid dipping and sagging
- Do not lift too high – the lumbar spine should not go into extension
- Ensure that both hip bones stay level to avoid the tendency to drop one hip bone below the level of the other hip bone as that foot lifts off the floor
- Maintain length on both sides of the waist to avoid shortening on one side
- Ensure the back of the neck stays long and the shoulders stay away from the ears

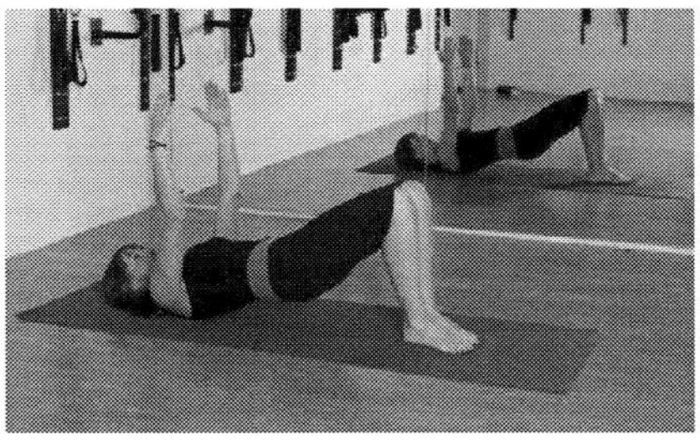

Variation Four

Variation One (Adaptation)

This exercise may be performed with just heel raises and no leg extension

Variation Two (Progression)

Once the knee has extended, hold it in the air, whilst performing ten butt squeezes on the supporting leg. Clench the buttock of the supporting leg up to ten times.

Variation Three (Progression)

Once the knee has extended, hold it in the air, whilst performing ten heel raises on the supporting foot

Variation Four (Progression)

This exercise may be performed with the arms held in the air, directly above the shoulders

Contra-Indications

Avoid "bridging" (i.e. arching the back by lifting the spine too high), as this will place stress on the lower back. In some cases, even a neutral position of the lumbar spine can cause discomfort. In these cases, the exercise may be performed with a posterior pelvic tilt rather than in a neutral position or avoided if discomfort persists.

Attitude in Mermaid

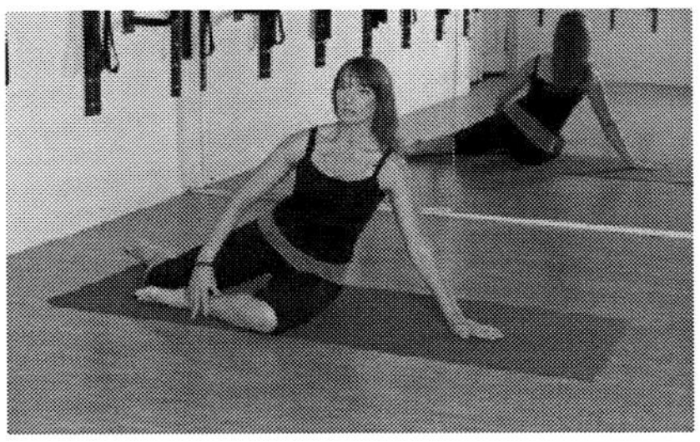

Aim

This exercise strengthens the gluteal muscles and the external rotators of the leg so requires good turnout

Starting position

Sit upright with the knees bent on the floor facing towards the right hand side of the body. Place the right hand to the right side of the body on the floor.

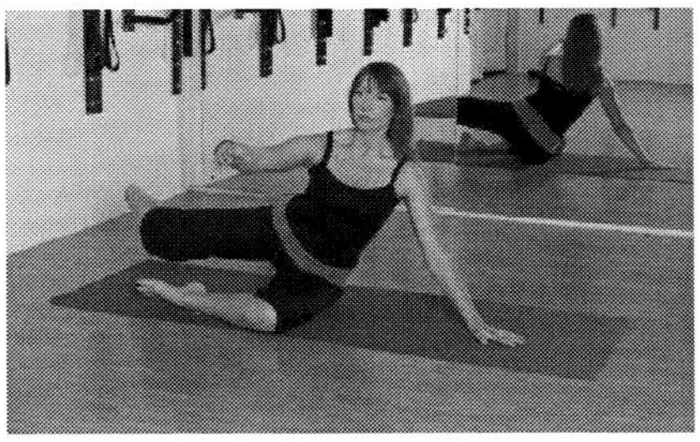

Action

Inhale – engage the core abdominals and lengthen up tall and raise the left arm up in front of the body at shoulder height and raise the top leg up off the bottom leg a couple of inches until the knee is slightly higher than the foot

Exhale – to engage the glutes and press the top thigh back behind the body a few inches, trying to keep the knee slightly higher than the foot if possible. The body remains as stable as possible, whilst performing small movements of no more than an inch in a pulsing like action

Repeat with the opposite leg

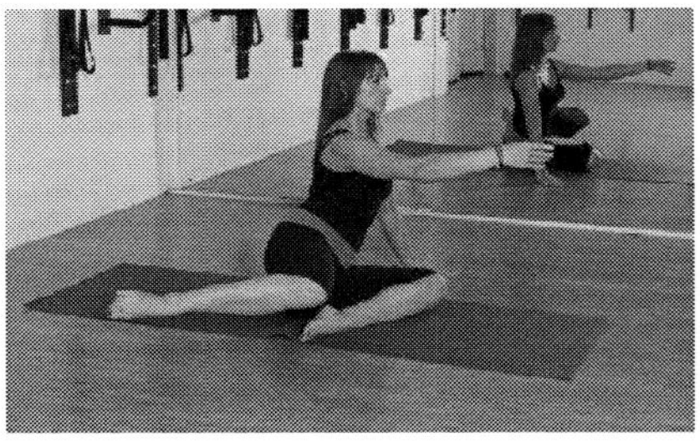

Target Muscles

Core abdominals, hamstrings, gluteals, lateral rotators

Watchpoints

- Maintain good scapula stability, with ears away from the shoulders
- Keep the external rotation of the leg throughout. If this is difficult, then limit the range of movement and height of the leg
- Use the core abdominals well so that the spine maintains stability
- Keep the hips, shoulders and pelvis as square and stable as possible
- Try to keep the knee higher than the foot throughout

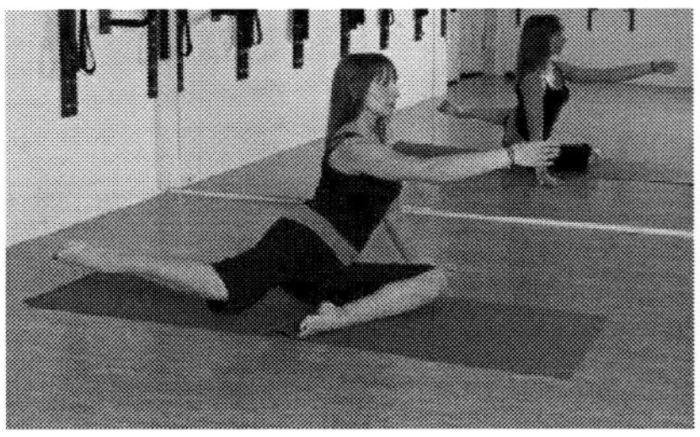

Contra-indications

A turned out position may not be suitable for those with sciatica

Torpedo

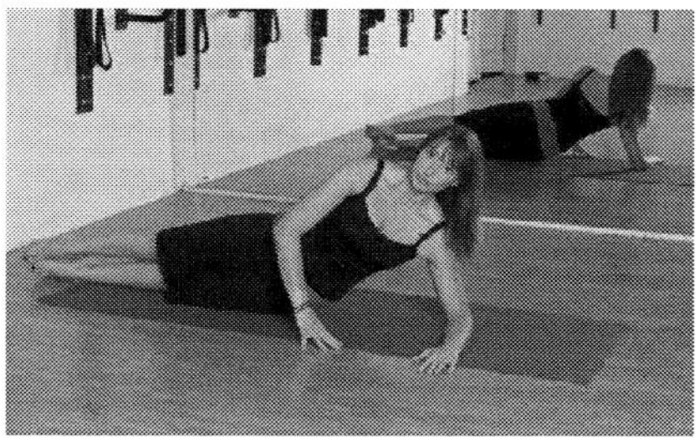

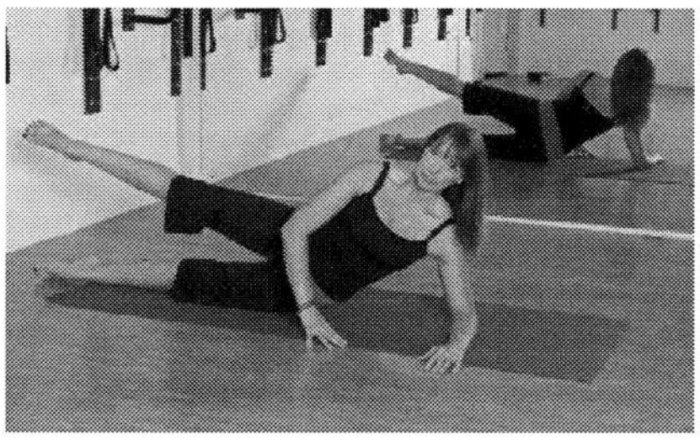

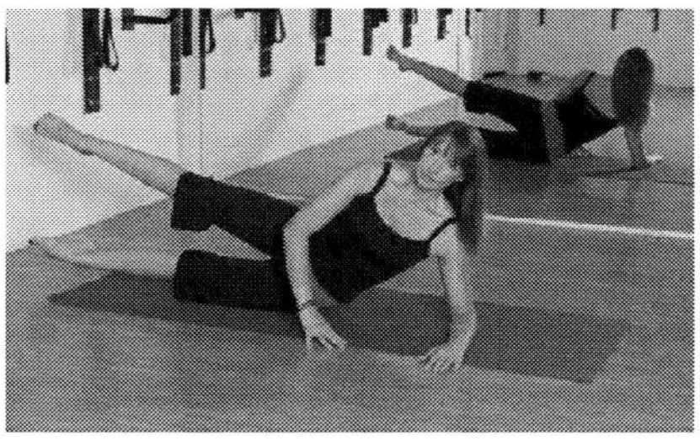

Aim

To work the inner thighs, whilst maintaining length in the waist and good pelvic stability

Starting Position

Lie on left hand side of the body with the left arm outstretched above the head. The right hand is resting on the floor in front of the body. Both legs are straight with feet, knee and hips stacked joint over joint and in alignment with the spine. Engage the core abdominals and externally rotate the legs out in the hip socket. Alternatively, the body may be propped up on the supporting elbow (as illustrated). Raise the top leg off the floor until the foot is a few inches higher than the hip.

Action

Exhale – Engage the core abdominals and lift the underneath leg upwards towards the top leg

Inhale – To lower the leg towards the floor without touching the floor.

Repeat with the opposite leg on the other side when finished

Target Muscles

Adductors, external rotators

Watchpoints

- Ensure the shoulders stay away from the ear and the gap between ear and shoulder remains equal on both sides
- Try to keep the length on both sides of the waist to avoid the tendency to shorten in the waist on the top side
- Keep the collar bones open
- Ensure that the hips are stacked joint over joint to avoid the tendency for the pelvis to roll back as the bottom leg lifts

Variation One (Adaptation)

This may be performed without both legs being in the air to minimise strain to the lower back. Bend the top leg and cross it over the bottom leg so that the knee of the top leg is bent at 90 degrees and rests on the floor. Raise the bottom leg as before.

Variation Two (Adaptation)

This may be performed in a parallel position.

Contra-Indications

External rotation may not be suitable for sciatica so choose Variation Two instead. Side lying exercises with both legs in the air can place extra strain on one side of the lower back. If discomfort is felt, then choose Variation one or avoid the exercise if discomfort persists.

Cross Stitch

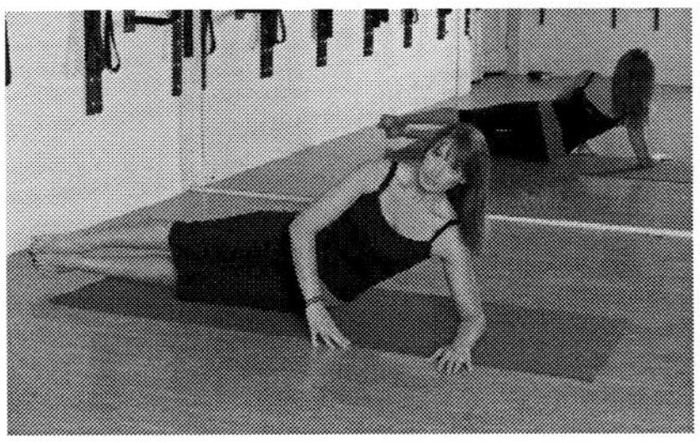

Aim

To work the inner thighs and external rotators whilst maintaining good pelvic stability

Starting Position

Lie on left hand side of the body with the left arm outstretched above the head. The right hand is resting on the floor in front of the body. Both legs are straight with feet, knee and hips stacked joint over joint and in alignment with the spine. Externally rotate the legs out in the hip socket. Raise both legs off the floor as high as stability allows. Alternatively, the body may be propped up on the supporting elbow (as illustrated).

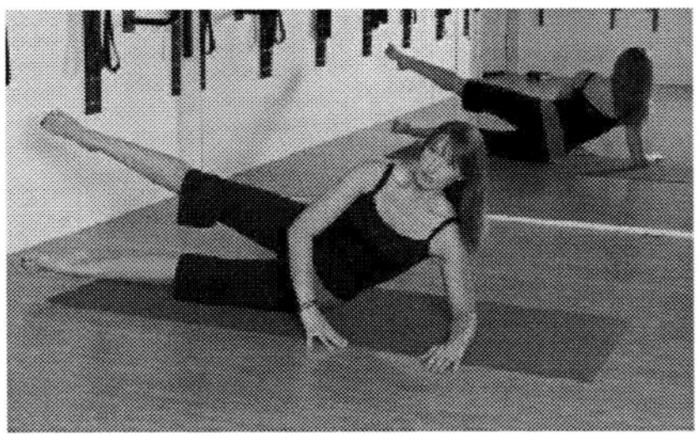

Action

Inhale – Engage the core abdominals and open out the legs a few inches. The top leg will raise higher and the bottom leg lower

Exhale – To bring the legs back together again but close the top leg behind the bottom leg so that the underneath leg is now in front

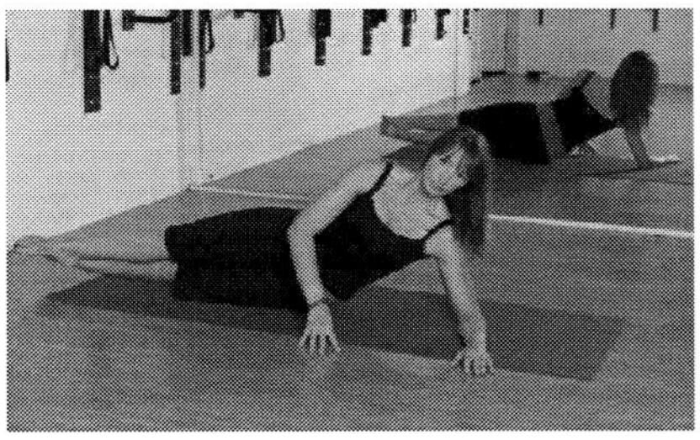

Inhale – Engage the core abdominals and open out the legs a few inches again

Exhale – To bring the legs back together again but close the top leg in front of the bottom leg so that the underneath leg is now behind again

Repeat on the other side when finished

Target Muscles

Adductors, external rotators, glutes, obliques, hip flexors

Watchpoints

- Ensure the shoulders stay away from the ear and the gap between ear and shoulder remains equal on both sides
- Try to keep the length on both sides of the waist to avoid the tendency to shorten in the waist on the top side
- Keep the collar bones open
- Ensure that the hips are stacked joint over joint to avoid the tendency for the pelvis to roll back as the bottom leg lifts

Variation One (Adaptation)

This may be performed without both legs being in the air to minimise strain to the lower back. Raise the top leg as before, opening and closing in front and behind the bottom leg, whilst the bottom leg remains on the floor.

Variation Two (Adaptation)

This may be performed in a parallel position.

Contra-Indications

External rotation may not be suitable for sciatica so choose Variation Two instead. Side lying exercises with both legs in the air can place extra strain on one side of the lower back. If discomfort is felt, then choose Variation one or avoid the exercise if discomfort persists.

Press Up Preparation (Box Push ups)

Aim

To work the upper body whilst maintaining core stability

Starting Position

Come to an all fours position with the knees bent directly under the hips and place the hands on the floor directly under the shoulders. The pelvis is in neutral.

Action

Inhale - To prepare

Exhale, - Engage the core abdominals

Inhale - To bend the elbows out to the sides and lower the head downwards towards the floor, only bending the arms as far as a neutral pelvis allows

Exhale - To straighten the elbows and push the body back up to the starting position.

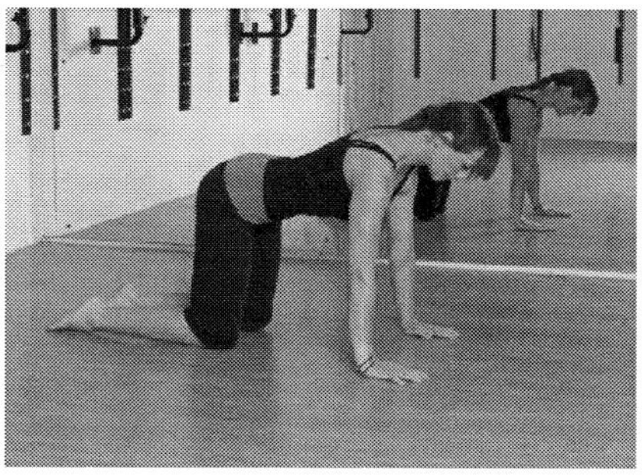

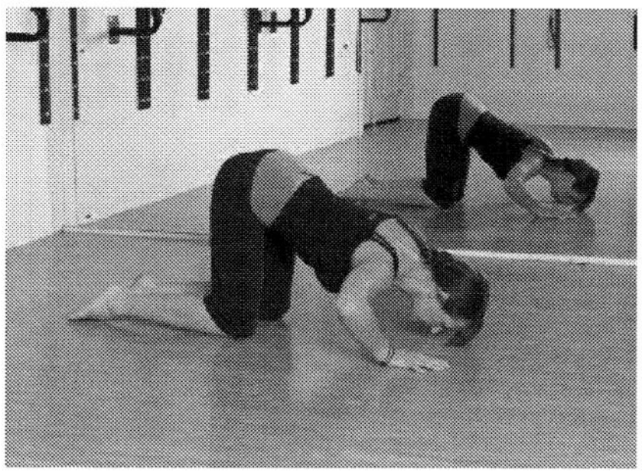

Target Muscles

Pectorals, anterior deltoid, triceps, core abdominals, serratus anterior

Watchpoints

- Ensure the core abdominals are engaged throughout to prevent the back from dipping
- Maintain the length between the ears and shoulders
- Only bend the elbows as far as a neutral spine can be maintained
- Try to avoid collapsing in between the shoulder blades. Engage serratus anterior to maintain the distance in between the shoulder blades
- The further forward the head is in front of the hands and the further forward the shoulders are in front of the hands, the more challenging (i.e. the body weight is forward of the hands)
- Try to keep the back of the neck long

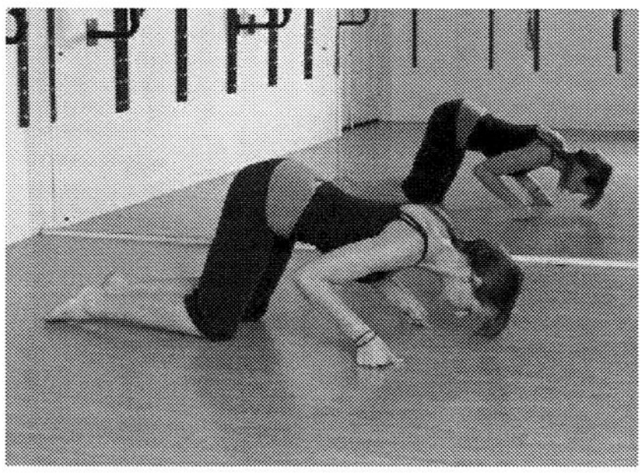

Variation One

Variation One (Adaptation)

To reduce pressure in the wrist joint, this exercise may be attempted on the knuckles of the hand, which will place the wrist in a more neutral position.

Variation Two (Progression)

The elbows may bend facing backwards (rather than sideways) in order to emphasise the triceps more. This is more challenging.

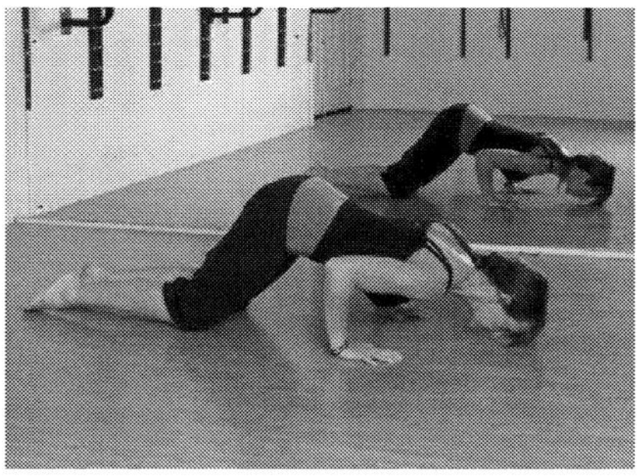

Variation Two

Contra-Indications

This exercise places extra stress on the wrist joints. Take extra care when attempting this exercise for certain clients with problems in these joints as it may prove unsuitable for them. Use Variation one in this instance.

Full Push Up

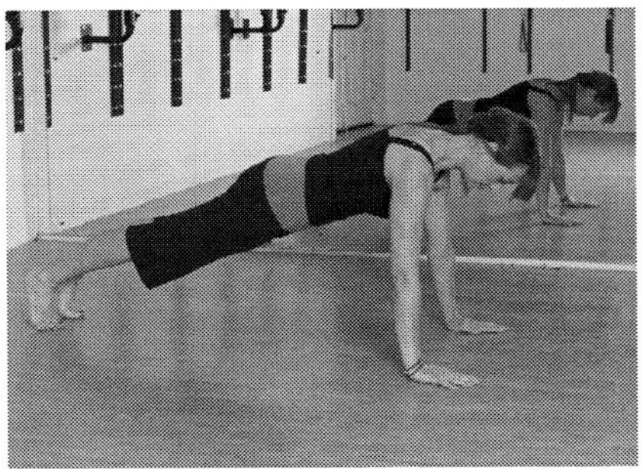

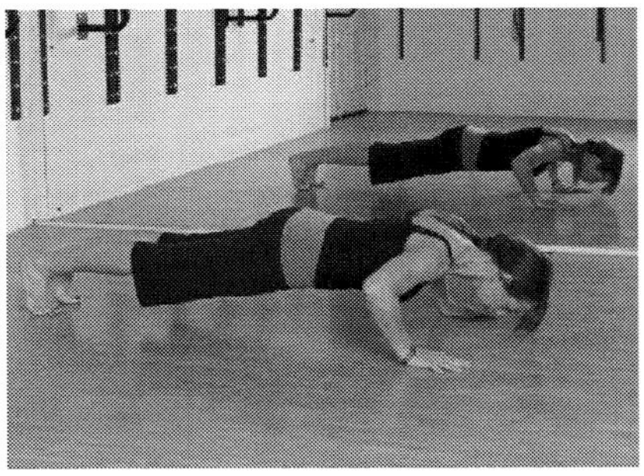

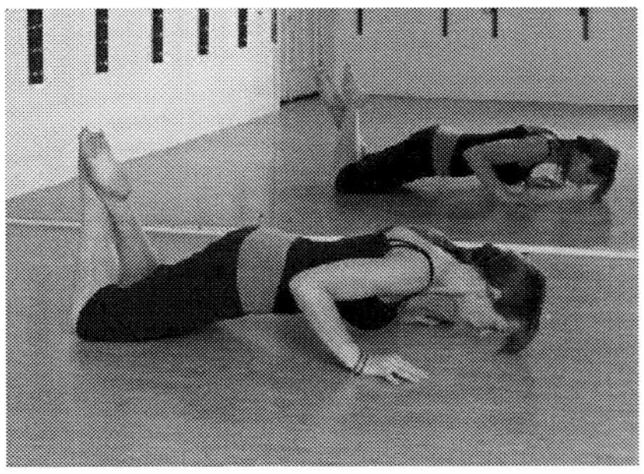

Variation Two

Aim

To work the upper body whilst maintaining core stability

Starting Position

Come to an all fours position with the knees bent directly under the hips and place the hands on the floor directly under the shoulders. Extend one leg at a time along the floor until the body comes to a plank position with the spine in a neutral position

Action

Inhale – To bend the elbows out to the sides and lower the body downwards towards the floor, only bending the arms as far as a neutral pelvis allows

Exhale - To straighten the elbows

Target Muscles

Pectorals, anterior deltoid, triceps, core abdominals, serratus anterior

Watchpoints

- Ensure the core abdominals are engaged throughout to prevent the back from dipping
- Maintain the length between the ears and shoulders
- Only bend the elbows as far as a neutral spine can be maintained
- Try to avoid collapsing in between the shoulder blades. Engage serratus anterior to maintain the distance in between the shoulder blades
- The further apart the hands are, the less challenging the workload

Variation One (Adaptation)

To reduce pressure in the wrist joint, this exercise may be attempted on the knuckles of the hand, which will place the wrist in a more neutral position.

Variation Two (Adaptation)

A three quarter press up may be performed (half way between a box and a full press up) as illustrated in the photo

Contra-Indications

This exercise places extra stress on the wrist joints. Take extra care when attempting this exercise for certain clients with problems in these joints as it may prove unsuitable for them. Use Variation one in this instance.

The Plank

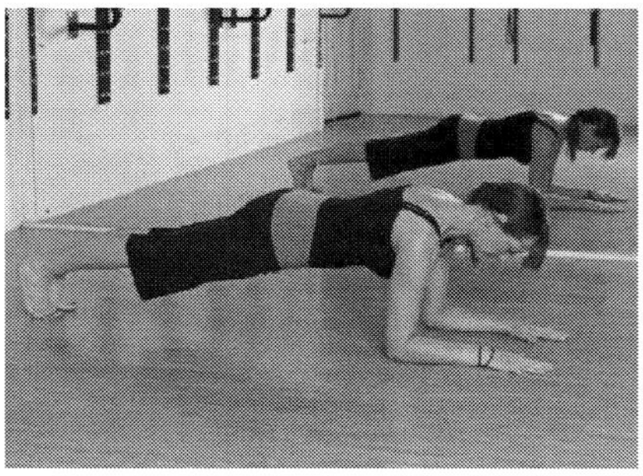

Aim

To strengthen the upper body whilst maintaining scapula and pelvic stability. Practice thoracic, lateral breathing.

Starting Position

Come to an all fours position with the knees bent directly under the hips and the elbows on the floor directly under the shoulders.

Action

Inhale -To prepare

Exhale - To engage the core abdominals and stretch the right leg along the floor until it is fully straight with the toes tucked under and then straighten the left leg along the floor until it is fully straight to come to a full plank position on the elbows, with the pelvis in neutral.

Hold this position for up to a minute, breathing in and out as normal. The abdominals must be held tight whilst breathing in and out to avoid sagging in the lumbar spine (i.e. thoracic breathing).

Target Muscles

Pectorals, anterior deltoid, triceps, core abdominals, serratus anterior

Watchpoints

- Ensure the core abdominals are engaged throughout to prevent sagging in the back
- Maintain the length between the ears and shoulders
- Try to avoid collapsing in between the shoulder blades. Engage serratus anterior to maintain the distance in between the shoulder blades
- Although the clock may be ticking for one minute, you may come in and out of position as many times as is necessary in order to rest, by bending the knees back to the floor for as long as you need to rest

Variation One (Progression)

Bend the right knee without allowing it to touch the floor. Repeat with the left. Alternate knee bends.

Back leg pull

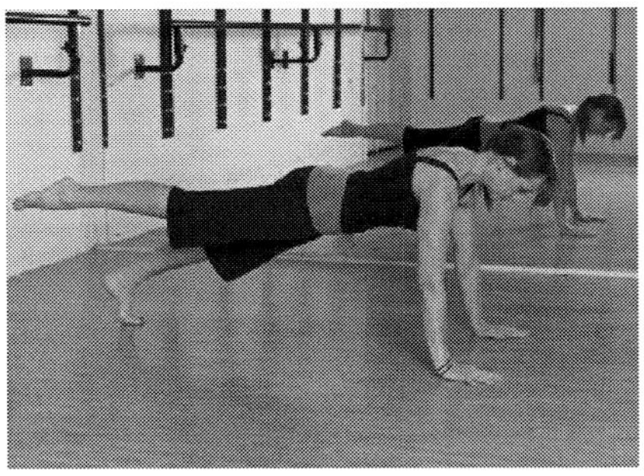

Aim

To challenge the upper body, maintain pelvic stability whilst raising a limb

Starting Position

Come to an all fours position with the knees bent directly under the hips and place the hands on the floor directly under the shoulders. Inhale to prepare. Exhale to engage the core abdominals, take the right knee off the floor and extend the leg straight out behind the body to rest on the tip toes. Repeat to raise the left leg until a full plank position is reached with the pelvis in neutral.

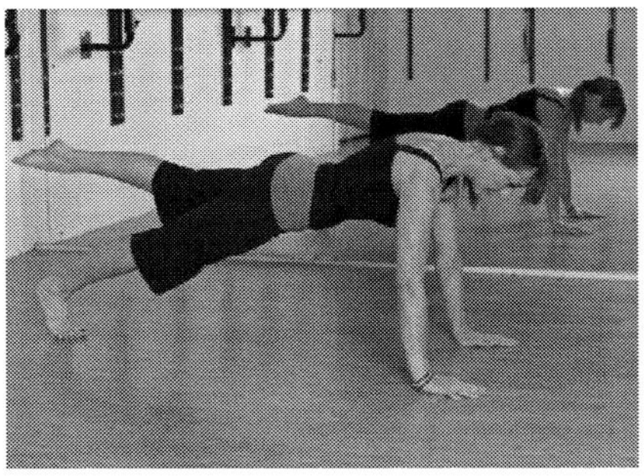

Action

Inhale - To prepare

Exhale - To engage the core abdominals, take the right foot off the floor and lift the leg straight up behind the body as far as a neutral pelvis can be maintained

Inhale - To return the right leg back down to the floor

Repeat with the left leg

Target Muscles

Pectorals, deltoid, triceps, core abdominals, gluteals, calves

Watchpoints

- Ensure the core abdominals are engaged throughout to prevent the back from dipping or the bottom sticking up as the leg lifts off the floor
- Maintain the length between the ears and shoulders
- Try to avoid collapsing in between the shoulder blades. Engage serratus anterior to maintain the distance in between the shoulder blades
- Maintain length on both sides of the waist
- Keep the hips and pelvis level throughout
- Only lift the leg as high as a neutral spine can be maintained

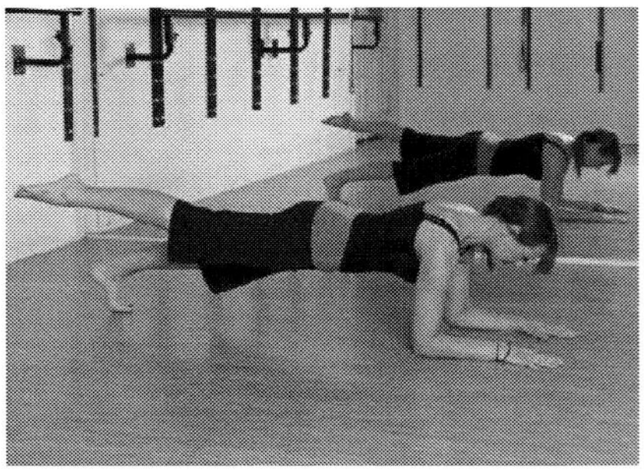

Variation One

Variation One (Adaptation)

This exercise may be performed on the elbows to reduce pressure in the wrist

Variation Two (Progression)

Once the right leg is raised, hold the position whilst the left foot dorsi flexes (i.e. perform a calf stretch with the left foot). Then plantar flex the left foot and return the right leg to the floor. Repeat with the opposite leg.

Contra-Indications

This exercise places extra stress on the wrist and shoulder joints. Take extra care when attempting this exercise for certain clients with problems in these joints, as it may prove unsuitable for them.

Plank Position – Lift opposite arm and leg

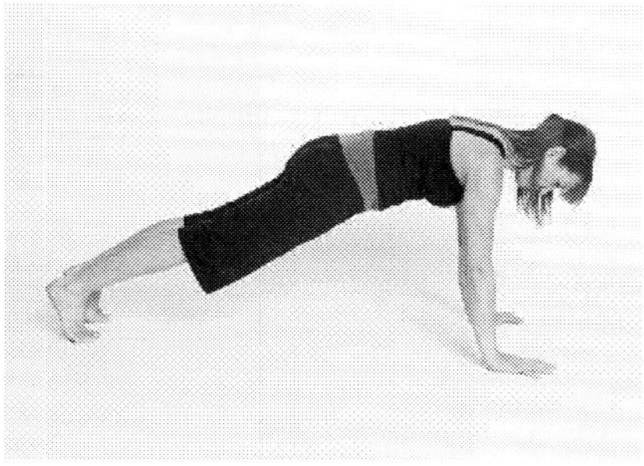

Aim

To challenge the upper body; maintain scapula and pelvic stability. Challenges co-ordination and balance

Starting Position

Come to an all fours position with the knees bent directly under the hips and place the hands directly under the shoulders. Inhale to prepare. Exhale to engage the core abdominals, take the right knee of the floor and extend the leg straight out to rest on the tiptoes. Repeat to raise the left leg until a full plank position is reached with the pelvis in neutral.

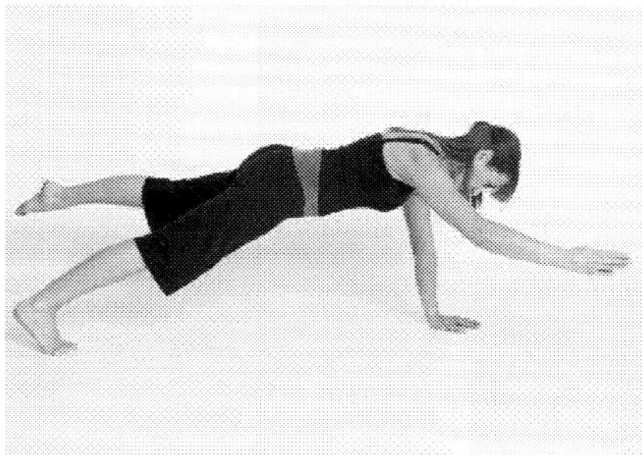

Action

Inhale - to prepare.

Exhale - to engage the core abdominals, take the right foot off the floor and extend the leg straight out behind the body as far as a neutral pelvis can be maintained. Simultaneously raise the left arm forward in the air until a tabletop position is achieved.

Inhale - to return both limbs back down to the floor. Repeat with the opposite side.

Target Muscles

Pectorals, deltoid, triceps, core abdominals, gluteals, calves, scapula stabilisers

Watchpoints

- Ensure the core abdominals are engaged throughout to prevent the back from dipping or the bottom sticking up as the limbs lift off the floor
- Maintain the length between the ears and shoulders particularly on the side that the arm lifts
- Try to avoid collapsing in between the shoulder blades. Engage serratus anterior muscle to maintain the distance in between the shoulder blades
- Only lift the arm and leg as high as a neutral spine can be maintained
- Maintain equal length on both sides of the waist
- Keep the hips and pelvis level throughout

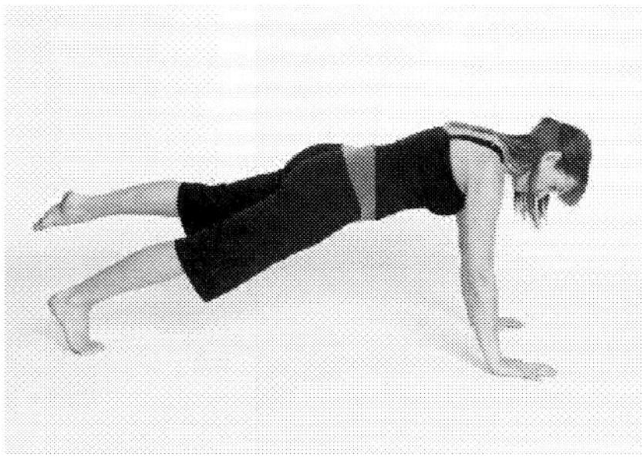

Variation One

Variation One (Adaptation)

This is an advanced exercise. Initially start with just lifting one limb. Alternate between lifting one leg, then one arm. When competent, try lifting both together.

Contra-Indications

This exercise places extra stress on the wrist and shoulder joints and may prove unsuitable for those with problems in these joints.

Side Plank

Aim

To strengthen the side of the torso and shoulders in this side plank position

Starting Position

Lie on the right hand side with the legs on top of each other in a straight line. The right elbow props up the body. The right shoulder should be directly above the right elbow with the forearm pointing forwards. The feet, knees and hips are stacked directly above one another. The left arm rests along the side of the thighs.

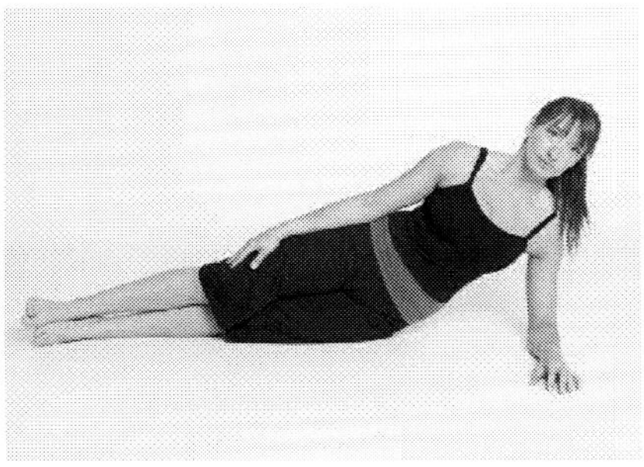

Action

Inhale - To prepare

Exhale - To engage the core abdominals and lift the hips and pelvis off the floor as high as the body allows. The feet and elbow remain on the floor. The left arm rises up in an arc overhead

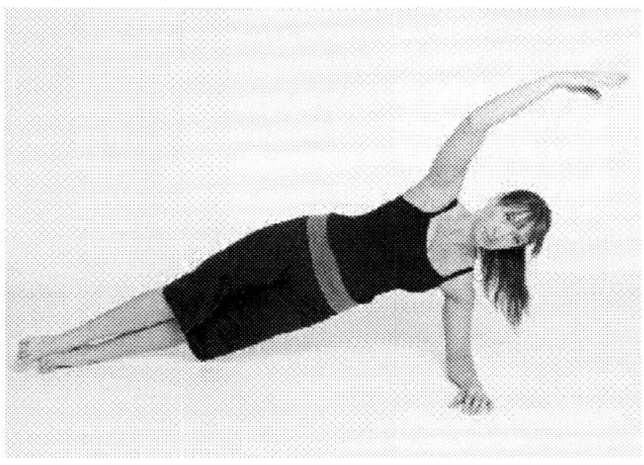

Inhale – To return to the starting position

Target Muscles

Quadratus Lumborum, obliques, deltoid, core abdominals, scapula stabilisers

Watchpoints

- Ensure good oblique engagement to prevent the bottom rib sticking out towards the floor
- Ensure good scapula stability to prevent collapsing onto the supporting shoulder
- Maintain the distance between ear and shoulder
- Keep the head in line with the spine
- Ensure that the elbow is directly under the shoulder at all times

Variation One (Adaptation)

This exercise may also be performed on the hand instead of the elbow

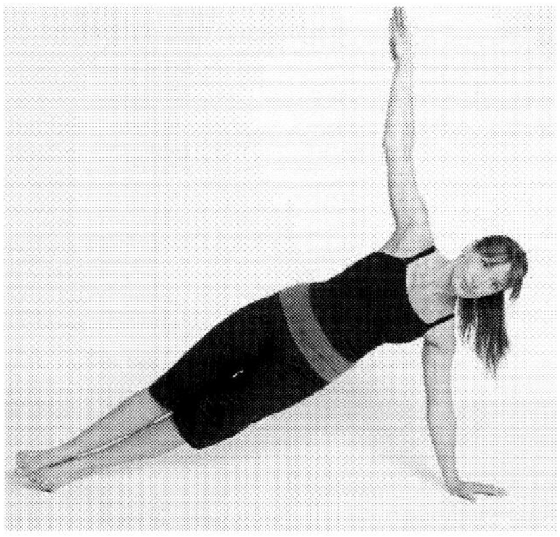

Variation One

Variation Two (Progression)

Inhale to raise the hips and then exhale to lift the top leg up off the floor. Keep the top leg slightly forwards on the lift otherwise the body tends to fall backwards. Inhale to place the leg back down and exhale to lower the torso to the floor.

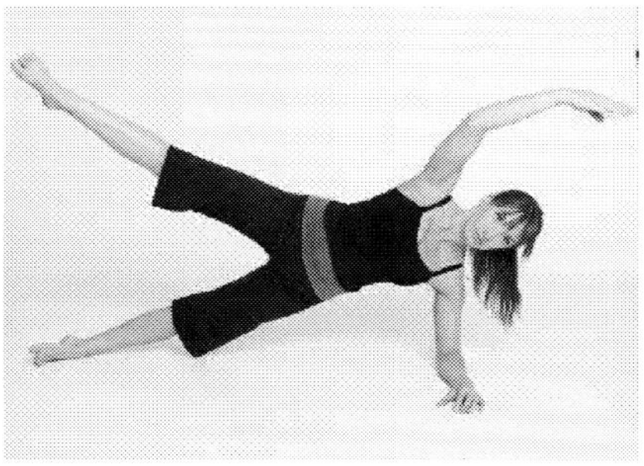

Variation Two

Variation Three (Progression)

Inhale to raise the hips and then exhale to twist the torso towards the floor. The left arm passes underneath the body and the head turns and looks behind the body to the right. Inhale to twist back around again and exhale to lower the torso to the floor.

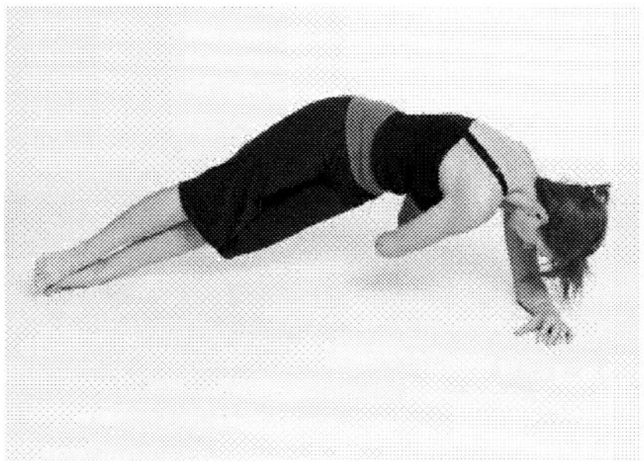

Variation Three

Contra-Indications

This exercise places extra stress on one side of the spine (depending upon which side is lifting) and this side may feel uncomfortable when performing this exercise so it may be unsuitable for certain back problems.

Oblique Plank

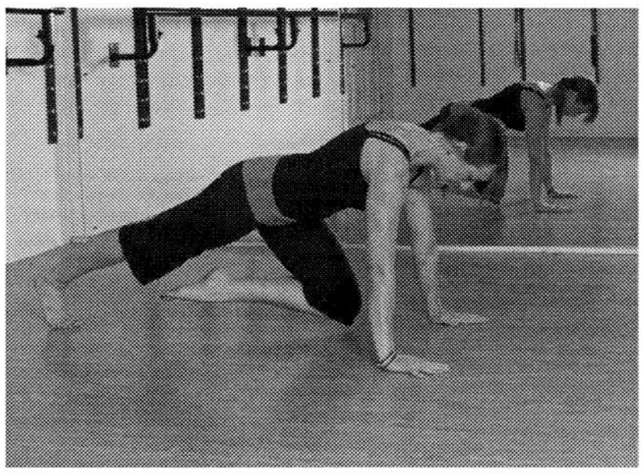

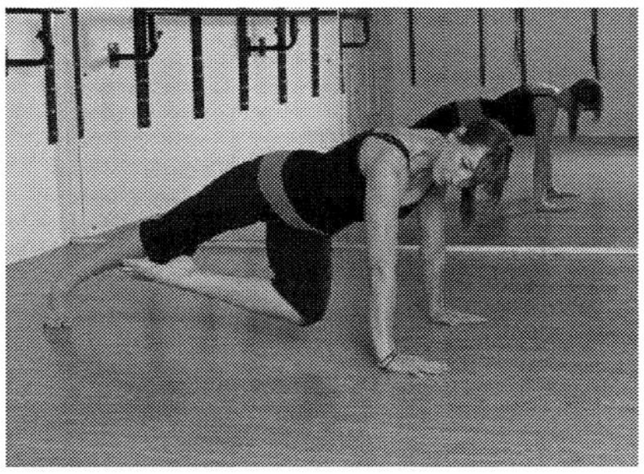

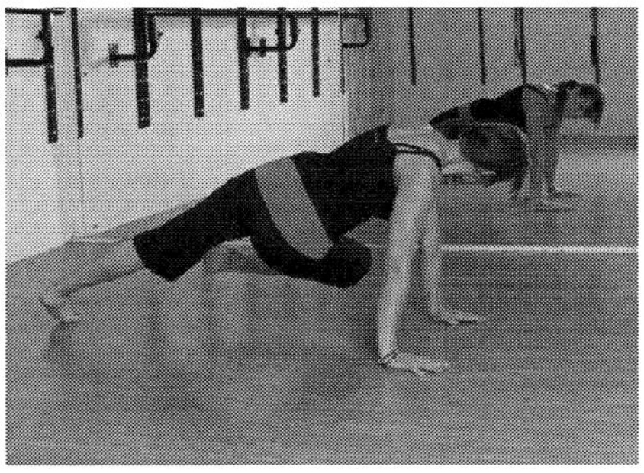

Aim

To strengthen the obliques and the upper body whilst maintaining scapula and pelvic stability. An extremely challenging exercise.

Starting Position

Come to an all fours position with the knees bent directly under the hips and the hands on the floor directly under the shoulders. Engage the core abdominals and stretch the right leg along the floor until it is fully straight with the toes tucked under and then straighten the left leg along the floor until it is fully straight to come to a full plank position

Action

Inhale –To take the right foot off the floor and bend the knee it towards the chest, whilst maintaining the buttocks at the same height

Exhale – Twist the spine and bring the knee across the body and over to the left, still keeping the buttocks at the same height

Inhale –To reverse the twist, bringing the knee back to the centre line. The leg may be straightened and lowered to the floor by way of rest initially but the aim is to string ten repetitions together before the leg touches the floor.

Repeat with the opposite leg

Target Muscles

Pectorals, anterior deltoid, triceps, core abdominals, serratus anterior, obliques

Watchpoints

- Ensure the core abdominals are engaged throughout to prevent sagging in the back
- Maintain the length between the ears and shoulders
- Try to avoid collapsing in between the shoulder blades. Engage serratus anterior to maintain the distance in between the shoulder blades
- Try to keep the hips and shoulders level and square as the spine rotates

Variation One (Adaptation)

To reduce pressure in the wrist joint, this exercise may be attempted on the elbows, which will place the wrist in a neutral position.

Reverse Plank

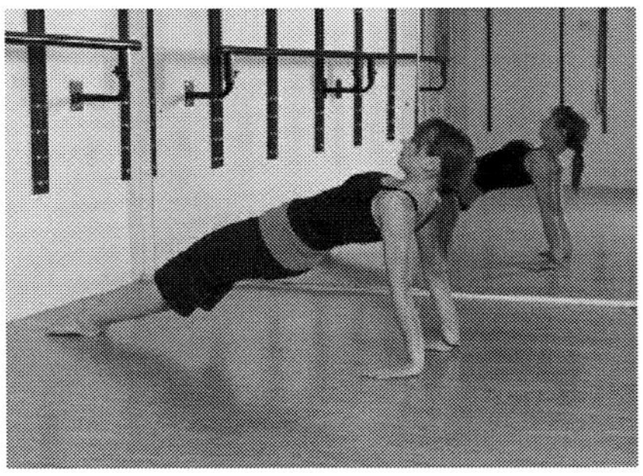

Aim

To challenge the upper body and maintain pelvic stability whilst raising a limb

Starting Position

Sit upright with the legs straight. The arms stretch backwards behind the body a few inches behind the buttocks. The palms are face down with the fingertips facing towards the body.

Action

Inhale - To engage the core abdominals and raise the hips and buttocks off the floor. Aim to make a diagonal straight line with the body so that the ankle, knees, buttocks and shoulders are aligned

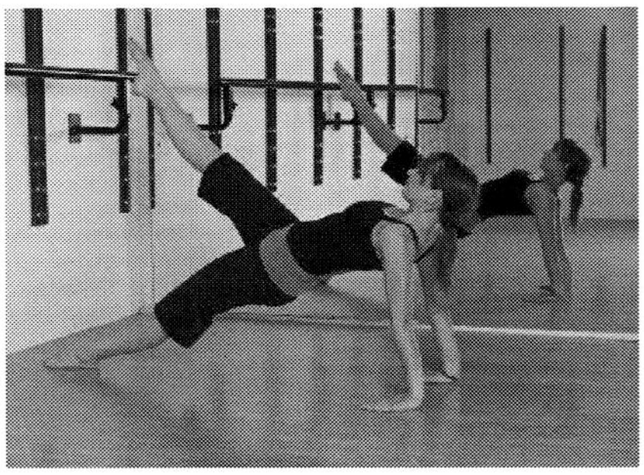

Exhale - Keeping the core abdominals engaged and take the right foot off the floor and extend the leg straight out in front of the body as far as a neutral pelvis can be maintained

Inhale - To return the right leg back down to the floor

Repeat with the left leg

Target Muscles

Pectorals, deltoid, triceps, core abdominals, gluteals, calves, hip flexors, quadriceps, hamstrings

Watchpoints

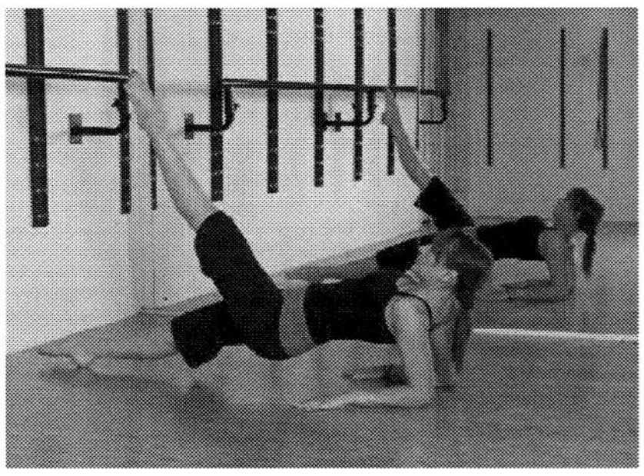

Variation Three

- Ensure the core abdominals are engaged throughout to prevent the buttocks from dipping or back arching as the leg lifts off the floor
- Maintain length on both sides of the waist
- Keep the hips and pelvis level throughout
- Maintain the length between the ears and shoulders
- Only lift the leg as high as a neutral spine can be maintained
- To reduce stress on the knee joint, the supporting leg may be slightly bent

Variation One (Adaptation)

To make this exercise easier, this may be performed with bent knees (reverse table top position)

Variation Two (Adaptation)

This exercise may be performed without the leg lift

Variation Three (Adaptation)

This may be performed on the elbows to reduce pressure in the wrist

Contra-Indications

This exercise places extra stress on the wrist, knee and shoulder joints. Take extra care when attempting this exercise for certain clients with problems in these joints as it may prove unsuitable for them. Choose variation three instead.

Dolphins

Aim

To strengthen the upper body whilst maintaining scapula stability

Starting Position

Come to an all fours position with the knees bent directly under the hips and bend the elbows and place them on the floor directly under the shoulders. Clasp the hands together to form a fist. The toes are tucked under. Inhale to prepare. Exhale to engage the core abdominals and lift the knees off the floor and straighten the legs as much as possible. The body will form an upside down letter "V" shape.

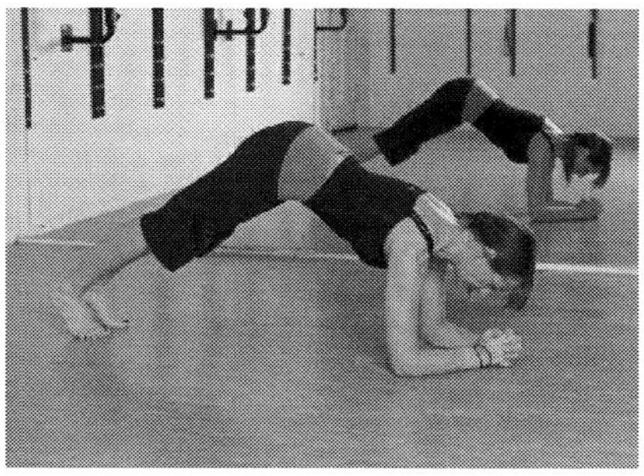

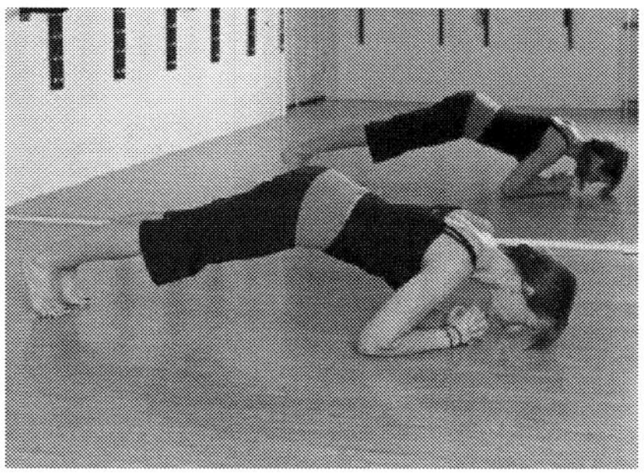

Action

Inhale – To prepare

Exhale - Engage the core abdominals

Inhale - To lean forwards and lower the body downwards towards the floor. (As the body leans forwards, the "V" shape will go wide, almost towards a plank position). You are aiming for the chin to touch the floor just in front of the fists if possible (or as close as the body allows)

Exhale - To push through the forearms, drawing the shoulders away from the ears and push the body back up to the starting position, maintaining core engagement throughout.

Target Muscles

Pectorals, anterior deltoid, triceps, core abdominals, serratus anterior

Watchpoints

- Ensure the core abdominals are engaged throughout to prevent straining the back
- Maintain the length between the ears and shoulders
- Try to avoid collapsing in between the shoulder blades. Engage serratus anterior to maintain the distance in between the shoulder blades
- The further apart the elbows are, the less challenging the workload
- The further away the feet are from the hands, the easier the workload for the upper body but the more challenging for the core

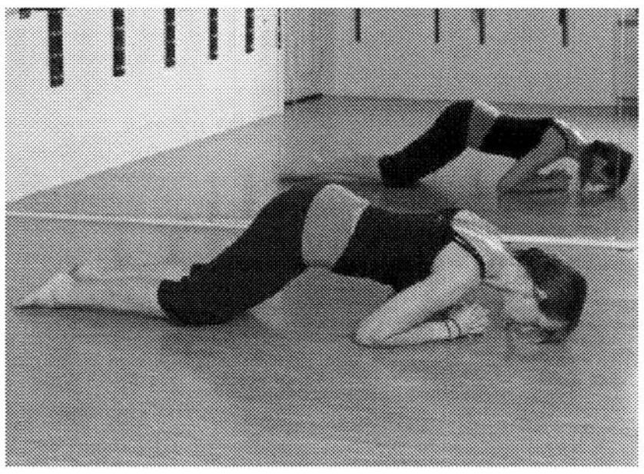

Variation One

Variation One (Adaptation)

This exercise may be done with the knees down on the floor to make it easier

Variation Two (Progression)

This exercise may be done with one leg back up in the air (arabesque). Alternate legs for each repetition

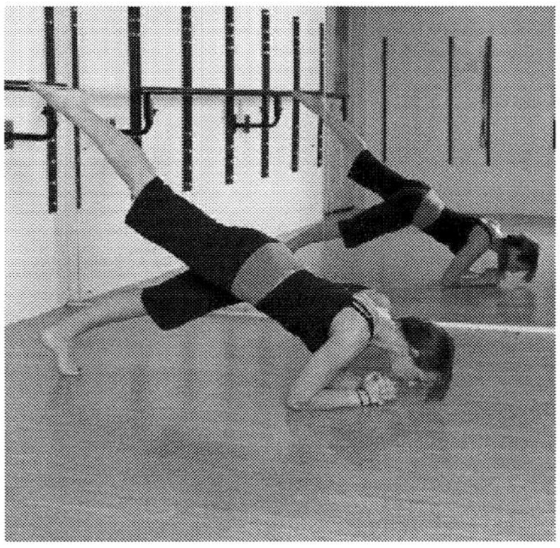

Variation Two

Tricep Press

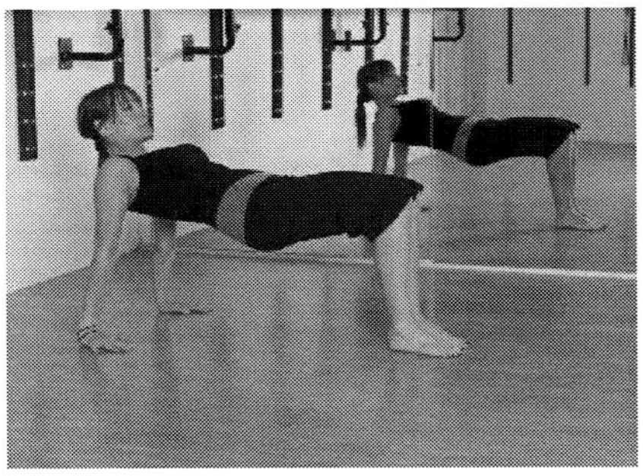

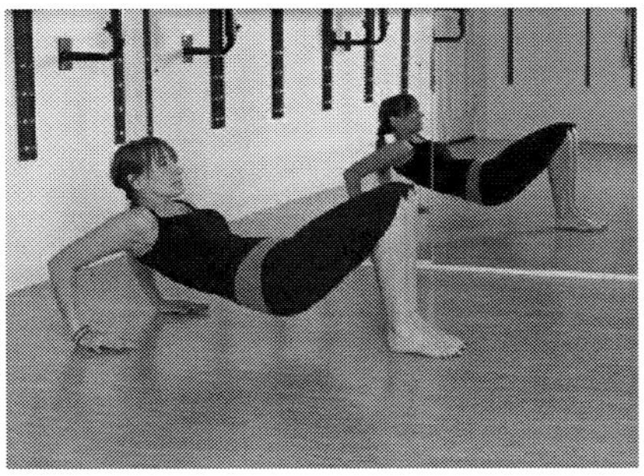

Aim

To work the triceps

Starting Position

Sit upright with the knees bent and the hands on the floor directly behind the buttocks. The arms are straight and the fingertips face towards the body. Raise the buttocks off the floor about ten inches (or wherever ability allows)

Action

Inhale - to prepare

Exhale - to engage the core abdominals and bend the elbows. As the elbows bend, the body will lower towards the floor

Inhale - to straighten the elbows and push the body back up to the starting position

Target Muscles

Triceps

Watchpoints

- Ensure the shoulders stay away from the ears and the back of the neck stays long
- Try to avoid collapsing in between the shoulder blades.
- Try not to use the legs to help push the body back upwards
- As the elbows bend, do not allow the buttocks to move towards the heels. The buttocks should remain in a constant position in space without deliberately lifting or lowering the pelvis to assist the movement
- Keep the elbows close together and pointing backwards to avoid them pointing out sideways

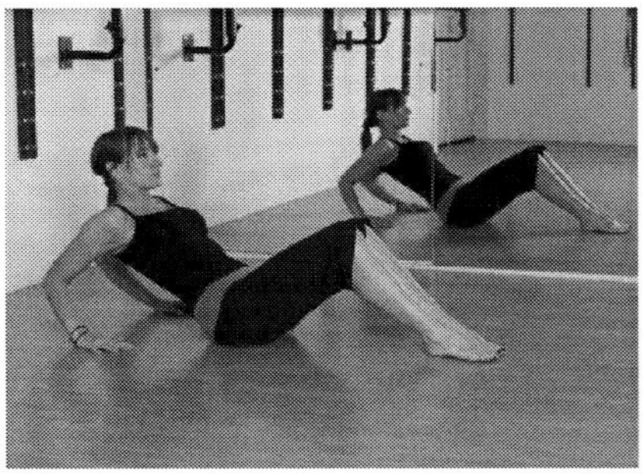

Variation One

Variation One (Adaptation)

This exercise may be done with the buttocks on the floor. The action is the same. Bend the elbows backwards and then try to get the body to resist when straightening the elbows.

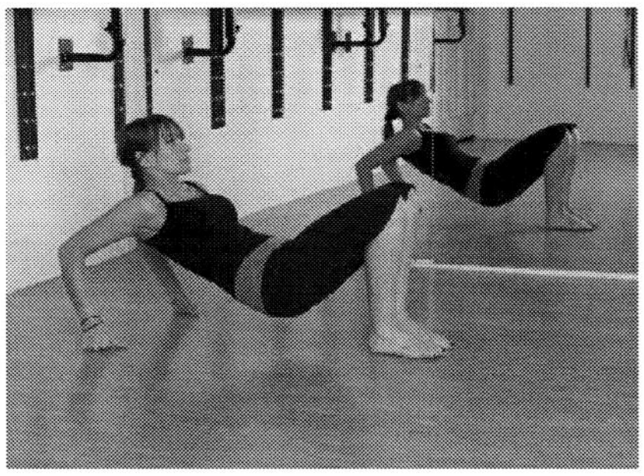

Variation Two

Variation Two (Adaptation)

This exercise may be done on the knuckles if there are wrist problems present.

Contra-Indications

This exercise places extra stress on the wrist joints. Take extra care when attempting this exercise for certain clients with problems in these joints, as it may prove unsuitable for them. Choose option two instead.

The Seesaw

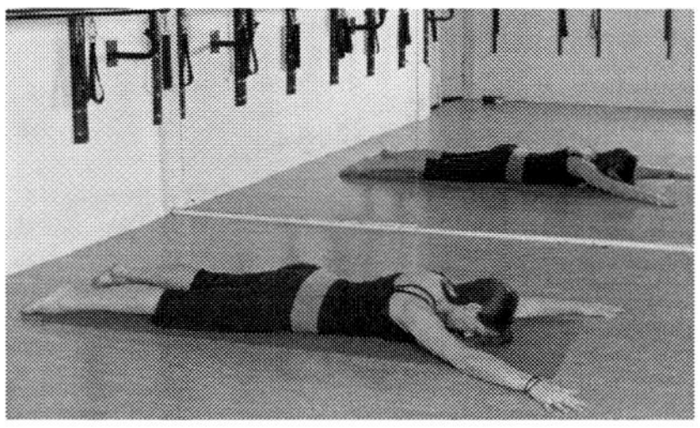

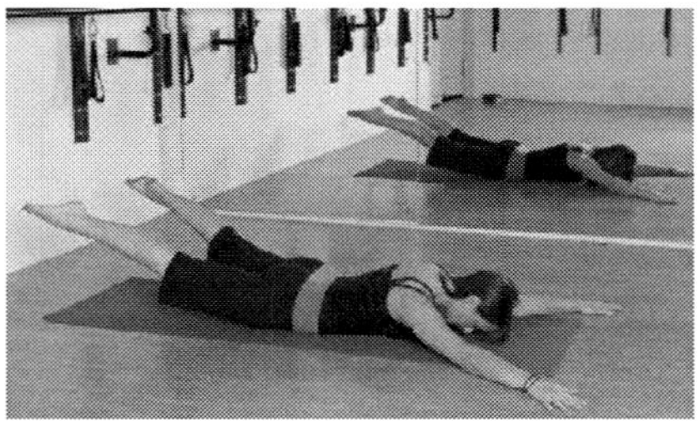

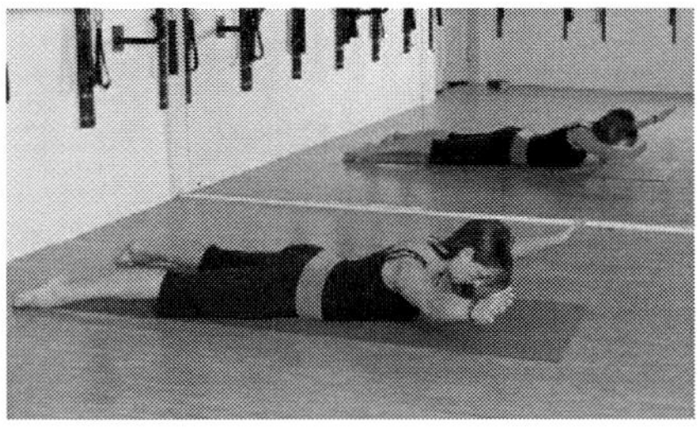

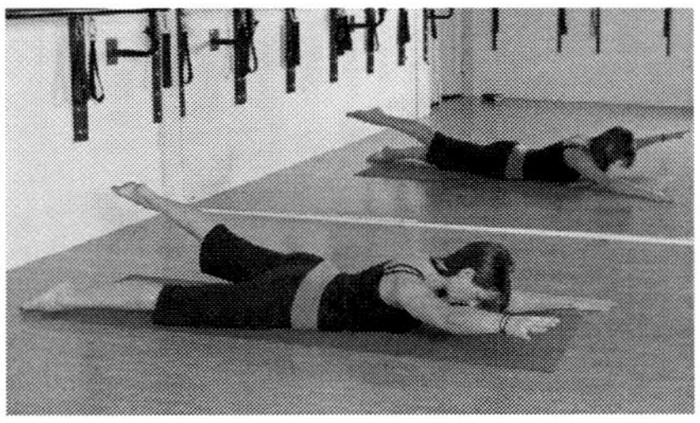

Variation One

Aim

To learn to work with opposition (i.e. lengthening whilst strengthening). To maintain good scapula stability and co-ordination.

Starting Position

Lie prone in a star shape with the arms and legs apart. A small head cushion may be placed under the forehead.

Action

Inhale - To prepare

Exhale - To engage the core abdominals and glutes and stretch both legs along the floor until they are as long as possible. Continue exhaling and lift the legs up off the floor.

Inhale – To lower the legs back down to the floor again

Exhale - To engage the core abdominals and stretch both arms forwards and away from the body without hiking the shoulders up to the ear. In addition, also lift the head and chest off the floor at the same time as the arms lift. The eyes are looking down to the floor so the back of the neck remains long

Inhale – To lower the torso back down to the floor again.

Alternate between lifting the arms and the legs

Target Muscles

Core Abdominals, gluteals, scapula stabilisers, erector spinae

Watchpoints

- Keep the waist long and even on both sides
- Keep the distance between ear and shoulder even on both sides to maintain good scapula stability
- Widen the arms to quarter to three (or lower) if scapula stability cannot be maintained
- As the limbs lift, ensure the body stays centred and does not rock over to one side
- Maintain a good sense of opposition against a strong centre
- Keep the back of the neck long

Variation One (Adaptation)

This exercise may be performed lifting opposite arm and leg to reduce strain to the lumbar spine

Variation Two (Progression)

This exercise should eventually be performed with a seesaw like action. As the legs lower, the arms simultaneously raise and vice versa. Therefore there is always one set of limbs in the air during the exercise.

Contra-Indications

Lying prone may be uncomfortable for certain back problems. Try putting a small cushion or rolled up towel under the abdomen to support the back.

Skydive

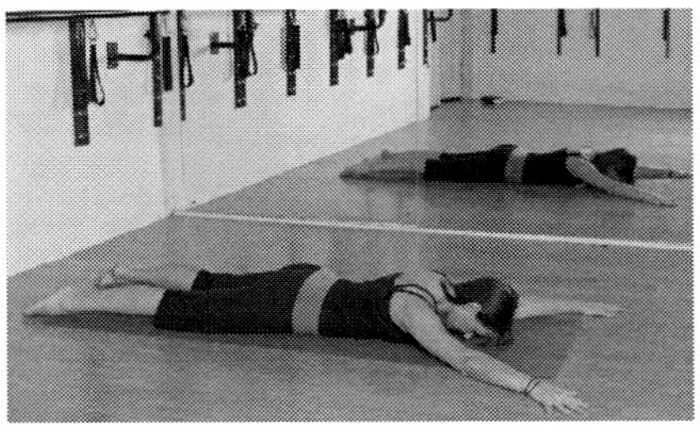

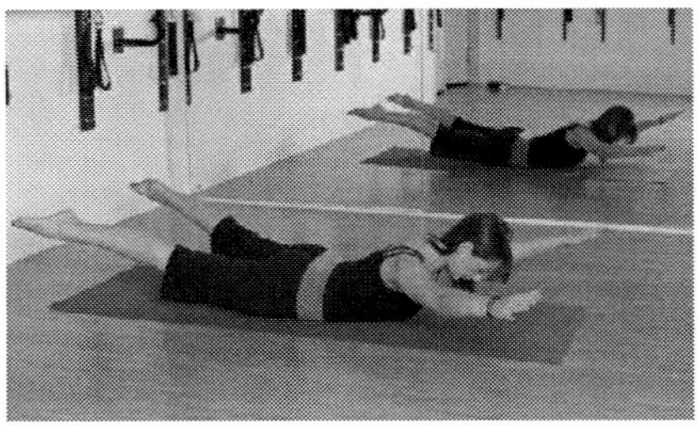

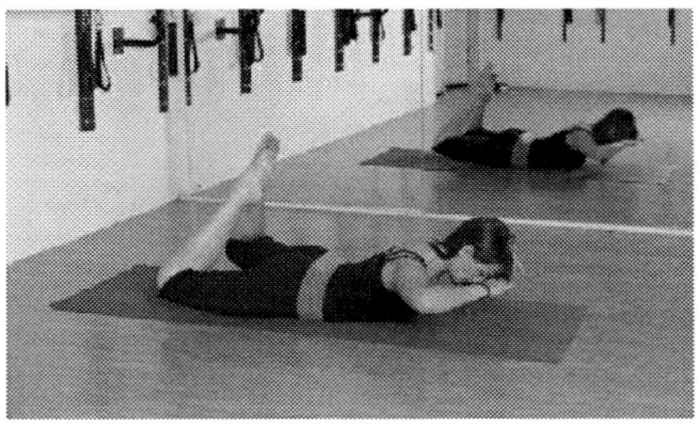

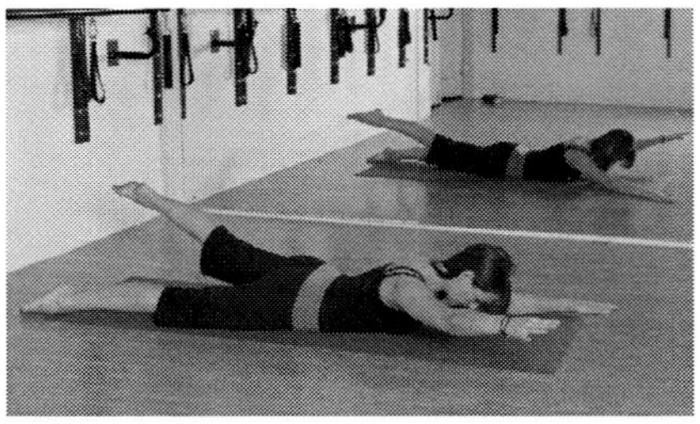

Variation One

Aim

To learn to work with opposition and control, whilst maintaining good scapula stability and co-ordination. This is a much more demanding exercise than the Seesaw

Starting Position

Lie prone in a star shape with the arms and legs apart. A small head cushion may be placed under the forehead.

Action

Inhale - To prepare

Exhale - To engage the core abdominals and glutes and stretch both legs along the floor and lift the legs up off the floor

Inhale – To bend the knees, bringing the heels towards the buttocks but keeping the thighs off the floor and the knees in space

Exhale – To extend the legs again, keeping the thighs off the floor and the knees in space

Inhale – To lower the legs back down to the floor again

Exhale - To engage the core abdominals and stretch both arms forwards and away from the body without hiking the shoulders up to the ear. Simultaneously lift the head and chest off the floor at the same time as the arms lift. The eyes are looking down to the floor so the back of the neck remains long

Inhale – Keeping the elbows in space, bend them and bring the hands to touch directly underneath the forehead with the palms facing down

Exhale – To extend the elbows again, bringing the arms back out to a star shape

Inhale – To lower the torso back down to the floor again

Inhale - To prepare

Exhale - To engage the core abdominals and glutes and stretch both arms and legs along the floor and lift all four limbs up off the floor

Inhale – To bend the elbows and knees, bringing the heels towards the buttocks and the hands under the forehead, whilst keeping the thighs and torso off the floor

Exhale – To extend all four limbs again, keeping the thighs and torso off the floor

Inhale – To lower the limbs back down to the floor again

Target Muscles

Core Abdominals, gluteals, scapula stabilisers, erector spinae, posterior deltoid, hamstrings

Watchpoints

- Keep the waist long and even on both sides
- Keep the distance between ear and shoulder even on both sides to maintain good scapula stability
- Widen the arms to quarter to three (or lower) if scapula stability cannot be maintained
- Keep the elbows and knees in space as they flex and extend

Variation One (Adaptation)

This exercise may be performed lifting opposite arm and leg instead, where all four limbs cannot be lifted

Contra-Indications

Lifting all four limbs may be unsuitable for certain back problems. Do Variation One instead or avoid if discomfort is felt. A small cushion may be placed under the hips to minimise discomfort.

Mid back series

Aim

This exercise strengthens the back muscles and stretches the spine.

Starting Position

Lie prone with the legs straight and the feet hip distance apart. The elbows are bent and the forearms are placed on the floor. The elbows are level with the shoulders and form a 90 degree angle (i.e. the hands are directly in line above the elbows). The head is resting on the floor and the chin is tucked in.

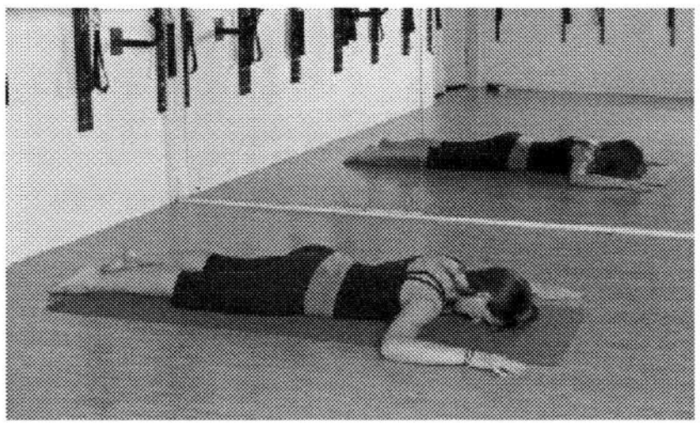

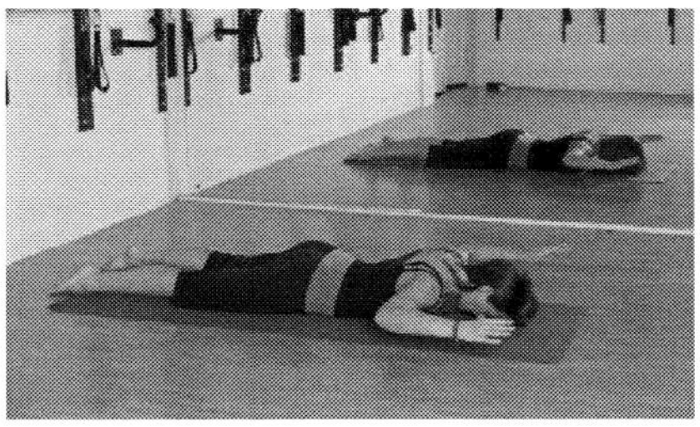

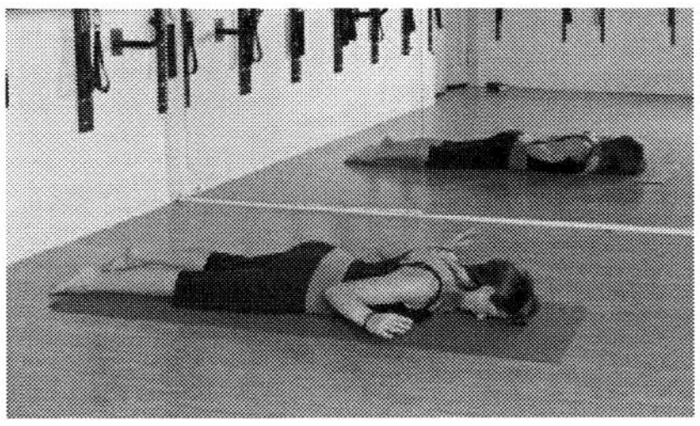

Action

Inhale - To prepare

Exhale - Engage the core abdominals as the scapula slide down the back. Maintaining a 90 degree angle, raise the arms off the floor as high as possible without hiking the shoulders up to the ears. Draw down the scapula, bringing the elbows slightly closer to the waist.

Inhale - To lower back down to the floor.

Target Muscles

Trapezius, neck extensors, scapula stabilisers

Watchpoints

- Ensure the scapula stabilising muscles are working hard to ensure that the shoulders stay away from the ears and the scapula stay apart
- Maintain good core engagement throughout
- Keep the back of the neck long and in alignment with the spine

Variation One (Adaptation)

Exhale to raise just the forearms off the floor but the elbows remain on the floor

Variation Two (Progression)

This exercise may be performed lifting the head and chest off the floor also

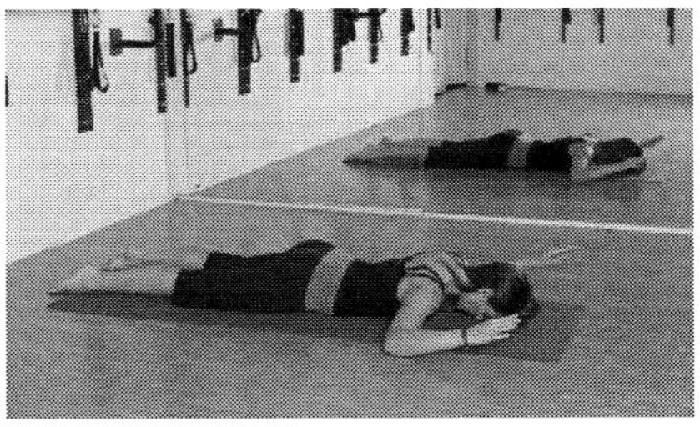

Variation One

Cobra

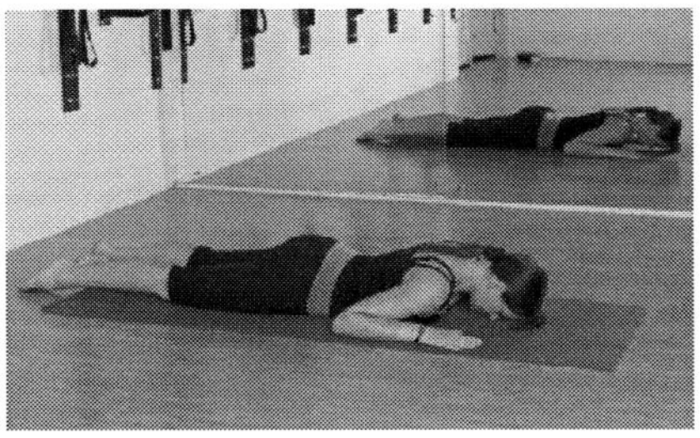

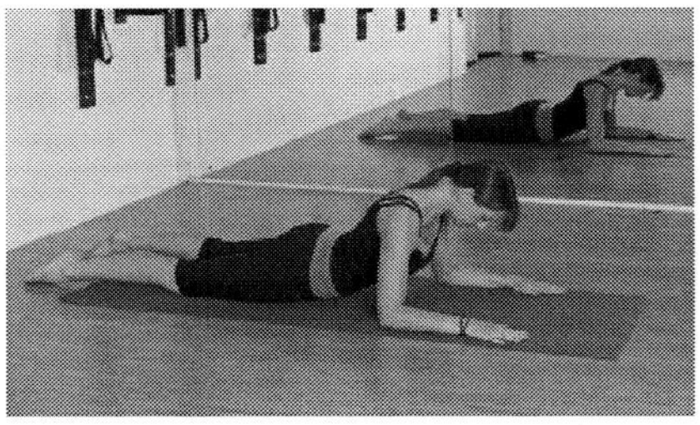

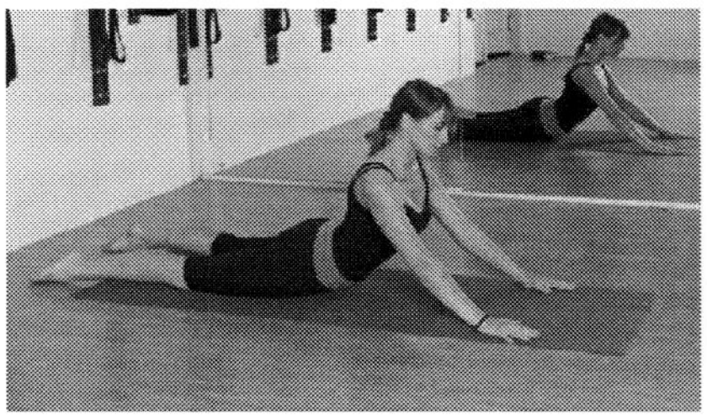

Variation One

Aim

This exercise strengthens the back muscles and stretches the spine.

Starting Position

Lie prone with the legs straight and the feet hip distance apart. The elbows are bent and the forearms are placed on the floor. The elbows are level with the shoulders and form a 90 degree angle (i.e. the hands are directly in line above the elbows). The head is resting on the floor and the chin is tucked in.

Action

Inhale - To prepare

Exhale - Engage the core abdominals as the scapula slide down the back. Imagine you are pushing away a marble with your nose. Slowly raise the forehead, nose and chin off the floor. Continue peeling the spine off the floor, vertebra by vertebra so that the chest raises a few inches off the floor. Ensure the last rib remains on the floor

Inhale - To lower back down to the floor.

Target Muscles

Back extensors, trapezius, neck extensors, scapula stabilisers

Watchpoints

- Ensure the scapula stabilising muscles are working hard to ensure that the shoulders stay away from the ears and the scapula stay apart
- Maintain good core engagement throughout
- Keep the back of the neck long and in alignment with the spine
- Ensure the 12th rib remains in contact with the floor. This is a thoracic extension not a lumbar extension.

Variation One (Progression)

Provided flexibility allows, a full lumbar extension may be performed. This may not be suitable for certain back problems.

Contra-Indications

This exercise may be unsuitable for certain neck and back problems if discomfort is felt whilst performing the repetitions.

The Eagle

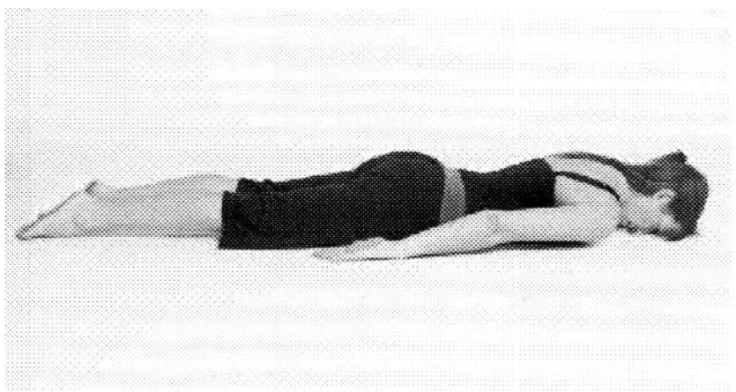

Aim

This exercise strengthens the mid back muscles and scapula stabilisers. The lats are much more involved in this version.

Starting Position

Lie prone with the legs adducted and the arms down by the sides of the body and palms facing upwards. Engage the core abdominals, open the collar bones and extend the thoracic spine a few inches off the floor. The hands lift off the floor with the palms facing inwards.

Inhale – To prepare

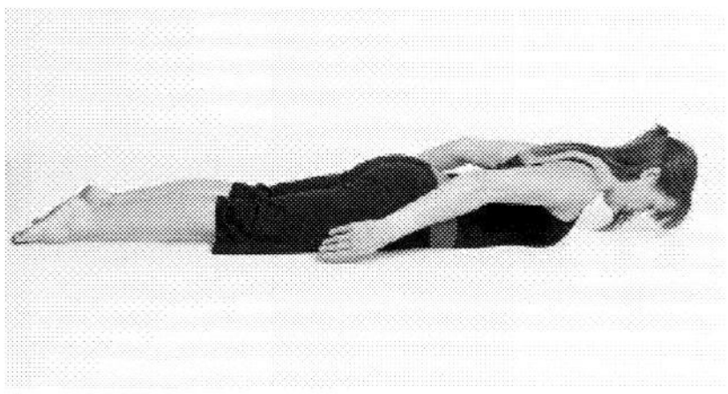

Exhale – To engage the core abdominals, draw down the scapula and open out the right arm to the side, aiming to get the hand at least level with the shoulder, if not a few inches further forwards, provided scapula stability can be maintained

Inhale – To draw the arm back in towards the waist

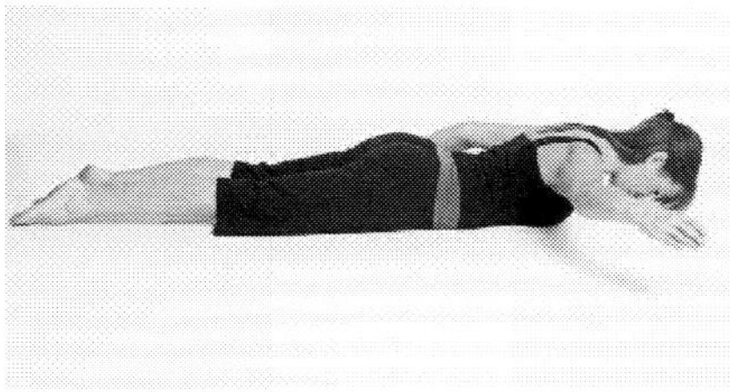

Exhale – To engage the core abdominals, draw down the scapula and open out the left arm to the side, aiming to get the hand at least level with the shoulder, if not a few inches further forwards, provided scapula stability can be maintained

Inhale – To draw the arm back in towards the waist

Exhale – To engage the core abdominals, draw down the scapula and open out both arms to the side, aiming to get the hands at least level with the shoulders, if not a few inches further forwards, provided scapula stability can be maintained

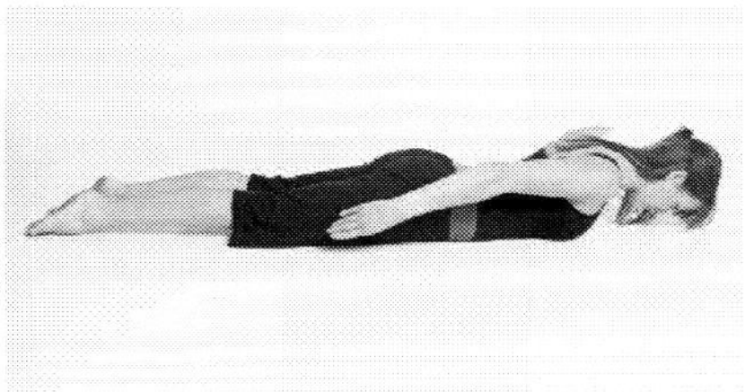

Inhale – To draw the arms back in towards the waist

Lower back down to the floor when the desired number of repetitions have been completed.

Target Muscles

Core abdominals, scapula stabilisers, neck extensors, posterior deltoid, back extensors, latissimus dorsi, teres

Watchpoints

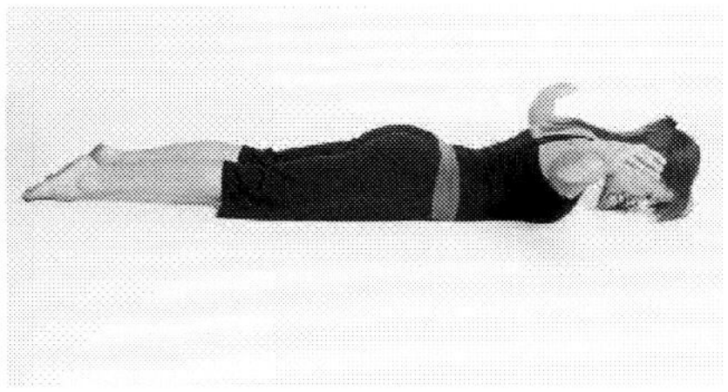

- Ensure the scapula stabilising muscles are working hard to ensure that the shoulders stay away from the ears and the scapula stay apart
- Maintain good core engagement throughout
- The range of movement at the shoulder joint should be limited to where good scapula stability can be maintained

Variation One (Adaptation)

This exercise may be performed without lifting the body off the floor.

Contra-Indications

This exercise may be unsuitable for certain neck and back problems if discomfort is felt whilst performing the repetitions. Try placing a small cushion underneath the hips to minimise discomfort or avoid altogether if discomfort persists.

Lean backs with chest press

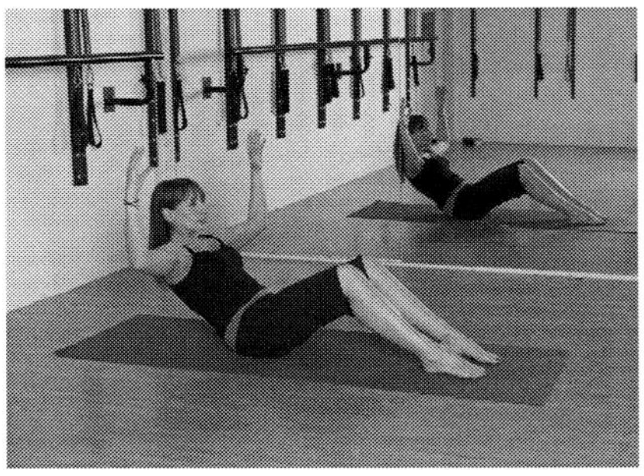

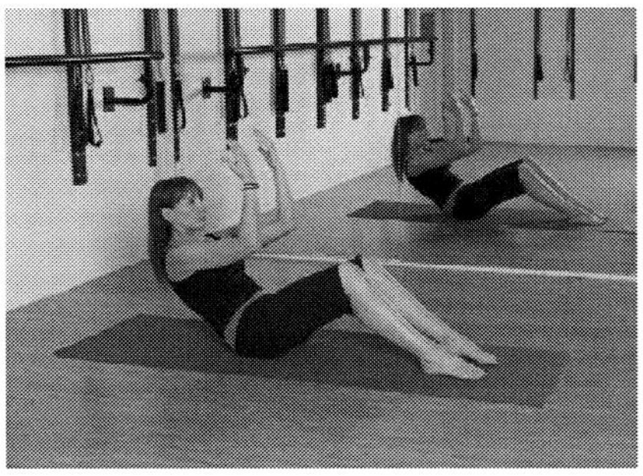

Aim

To work the abdominals and maintain an even C-curve in the spine

Starting Position

Sit upright with knees bent and feet on the floor, hip width apart. The arms are outstretched to the side at shoulder height with the elbows bent at 90 degrees. Ideally the spine will be in neutral (depending upon flexibility).

Action

Inhale - to prepare

Exhale – Engage the core abdominals and tilt the pelvis into a posterior tilt and roll backwards, one vertebra at a time as far as the body allows, maintaining lumbar flexion. Simultaneously bring the arms forwards in front of the chest so that the elbows are at shoulder height and in line with the nipple.

Inhale – to roll back up to the starting position, opening the arms again.

Target Muscles

Core abdominals, hip flexors, pectorals

Watchpoints

- Ensure that a degree of lumbar flexion remains throughout so only lean back as far as this can be maintained to avoid the lumbar spine going into extension
- Ensure that the feet remain on the floor
- Try to achieve an even curve throughout the spine so a not to over-flex the lumbar or thoracic spine
- Ensure the shoulders stay away from the ears
- Try not to grip around the hip flexors

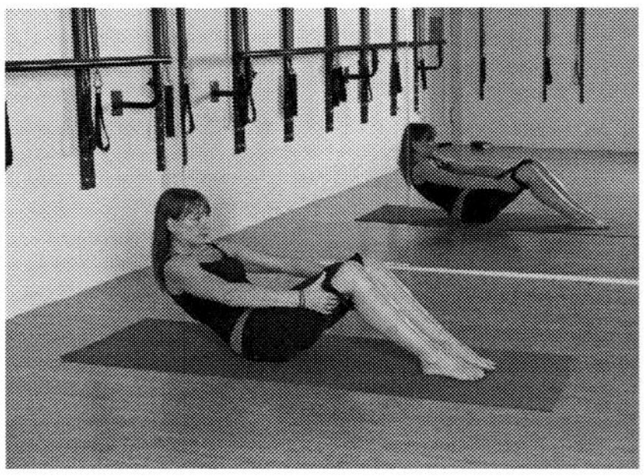

Variation One

Variation One (Adaptation)

Lean back with the hands behind the thighs for extra support

Contra-Indications

Lean back exercises may not be suitable for certain back problems

Lean backs with arm release

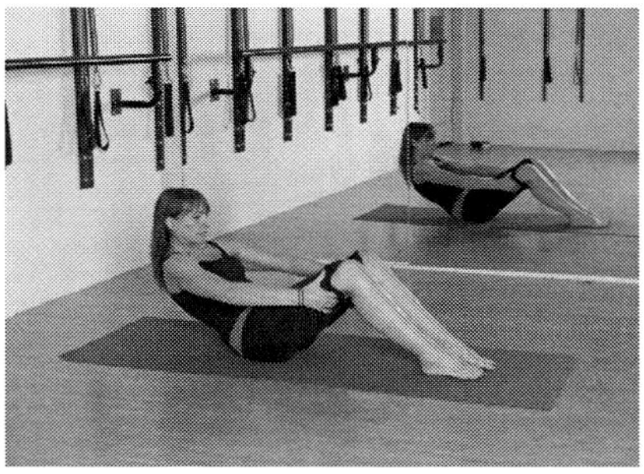

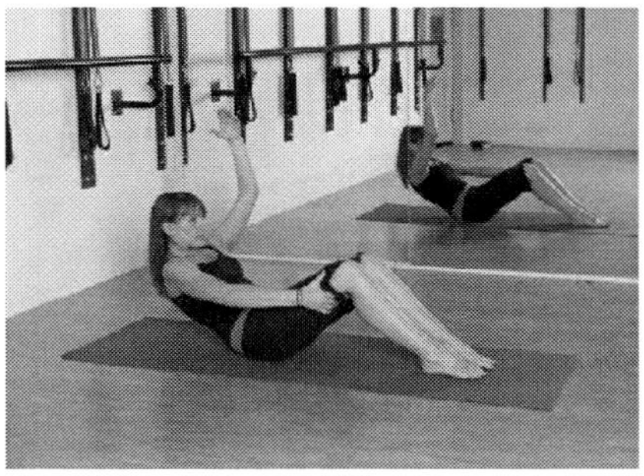

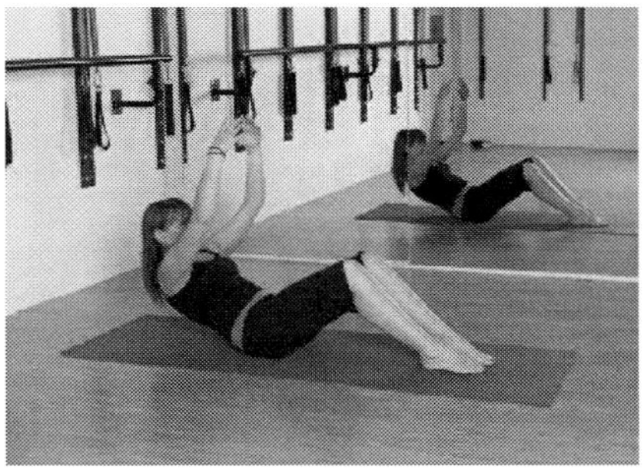

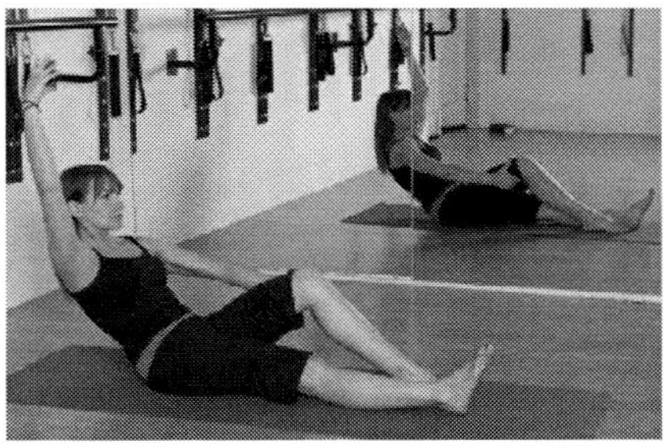

Variation Two

Aim

To work the abdominals and maintain an even C-curve in the spine

Starting Position

Sit upright with knees bent and feet on the floor, hip width apart. The arms are outstretched in front of the body and the hands are holding gently behind the thighs

Inhale - to prepare

Exhale – Engage the core abdominals and tilt the pelvis into a posterior tilt and roll backwards, one vertebra at a time as far as the body allows, maintaining lumbar flexion.

Inhale – to prepare

Exhale – to release one hand for a count of ten, bringing it above the head and breathing normally throughout
roll back up to the starting positions and open out the arms again.

Inhale – to lower the arm down amd place it behind the thigh again

Exhale – to release the opposite hand for a count of ten, bringing it above the head and breathing normally throughout

Inhale – to lower the arm down amd place it behind the thigh again

Exhale – to release both hands for a count of ten, bringing them above the head and breathing normally throughout

Inhale – to lower both arms down and place them behind the thighs and roll back up to the starting position when finished

Target Muscles

Core abdominals

Watchpoints

- Ensure that a degree of lumbar flexion remains throughout so only lean back as far as this can be maintained to avoid the lumbar spine going into extension
- Ensure that the feet remain on the floor
- Try to achieve an even curve throughout the spine so as not to over-flex the lumbar or thoracic spine
- Ensure the shoulders stay away from the ears

Variation One (Adaptation)

Lean back keeping the hands behind the thighs for extra support

Variation Two (Progression)

The above sequence may be done with one leg straight and the other leg bent

Contra-Indications

Lean back exercises may not be suitable for certain back problems

Oblique Lean backs

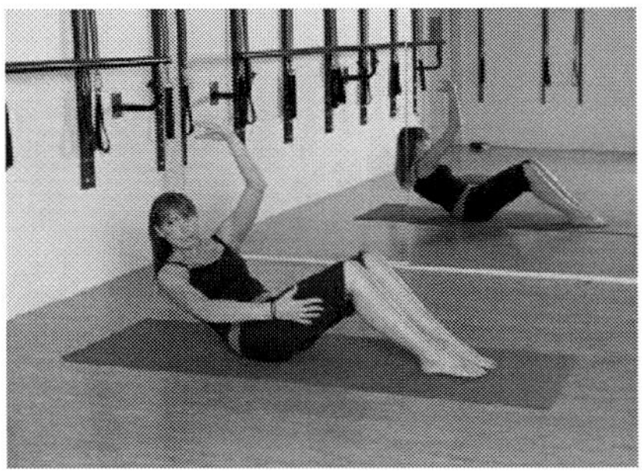

Aim

To work the oblique abdominals

Starting Position

Sit upright with knees bent and feet on the floor, hip width apart. The arms are outstretched in front of the body and the hands are holding gently behind the thighs

Action

Inhale - to prepare

Exhale – Engage the core abdominals and tilt the pelvis into a posterior tilt and roll backwards, one vertebra at a time as far as the body allows, maintaining lumbar flexion.

Inhale – to prepare

Exhale – to release the right hand, bringing it above the head, whilst keeping the left hand behind the left knee. Simultaneously oblique twist the torso over to the left

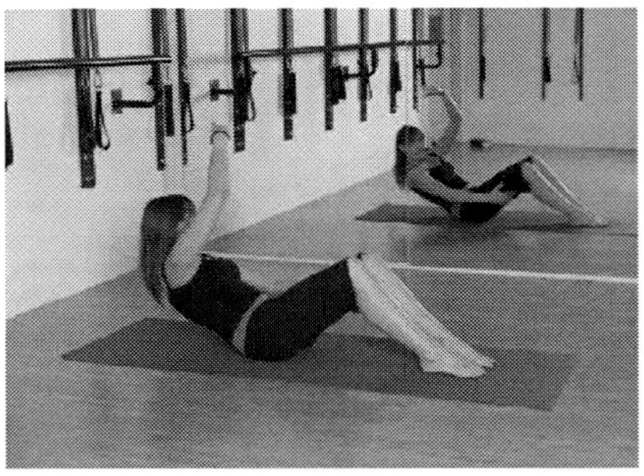

Inhale – to prepare

Exhale – to perform ten little contractions, pulsing no more than one or two inches of movement, increasing spinal flexion and rotation as well as abdominal contraction on each exhalation.

Repeat to the opposite side

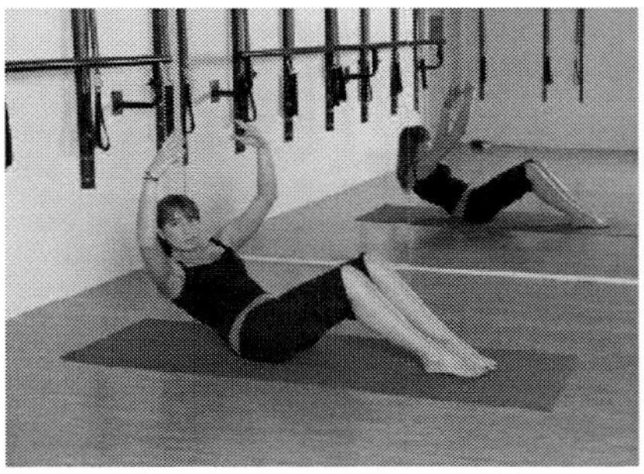

Variation Two

Target Muscles

Core abdominals, obliques, hip flexors

Watchpoints

- Ensure that a degree of lumbar flexion remains throughout so only lean back as far as this can be maintained to avoid the lumbar spine going into extension
- Ensure that the feet remain on the floor
- Try to achieve an even curve throughout the spine so a not to over-flex the lumbar or thoracic spine
- Ensure the shoulders stay away from the ears

Variation One (Adaptation)

Lean back keeping the hands behind the thighs for extra support

Variation Two (Progression)

The above sequence may be done with both arms in the air

Contra-Indications

Lean back exercises may not be suitable for certain back problems

Can Can

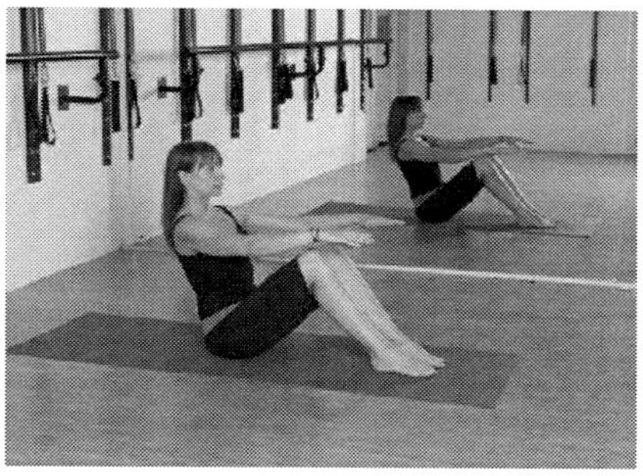

Aim

To work the obliques, whilst maintaining an upright posture and minimising the work in the arms

Starting Position

Sit upright with knees bent and feet on the floor, hip width apart. The arms are outstretched at shoulder height. Ideally the spine will be in neutral (depending upon flexibility). Engage the core abdominals and tilt the pelvis into a posterior tilt and roll backwards, one vertebra at a time as far as the body allows, maintaining lumbar flexion. The arms are outstretched in front of the body at shoulder height.

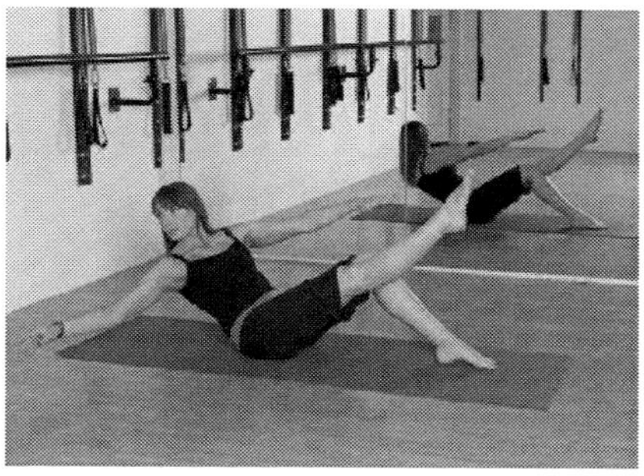

Action

Inhale - to prepare

Exhale - to engage the core abdominals and twist the torso across to the right. The right arm opens out to the side, whilst the left arm remains forward. Simultaneously straighten the right knee but keep the knees glued together as the leg extends.

Repeat to the opposite side

Target Muscles

Core abdominals, obliques, hip flexors, quadriceps

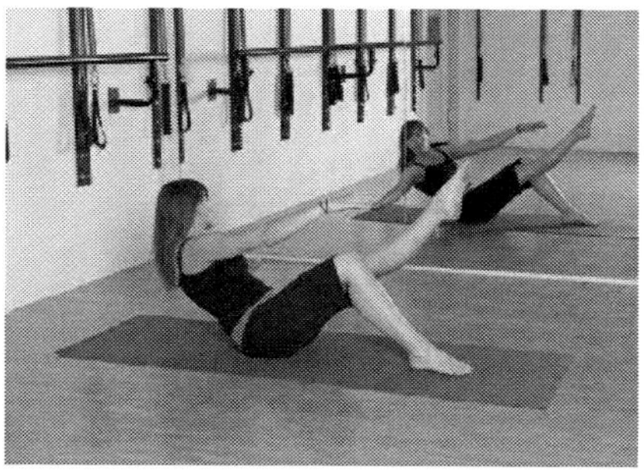

Watchpoints

- Maintain an equal length on both sides of the waist
- Ensure an equal pressure through both sit bones
- Ensure an equal length between the ears and shoulders on each side
- Ensure that a degree of lumbar flexion remains throughout so only lean back as far as this can be maintained to avoid the lumbar spine going into extension
- Ensure that the feet remain on the floor
- Try to achieve an even curve throughout the spine so as not to over-flex the lumbar or thoracic spine

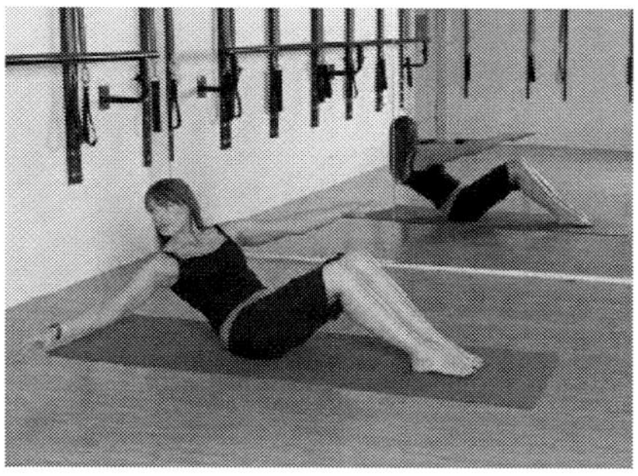

Variation One

Variation One (Adaptation)

This may be performed without the leg raise

Contra-Indications

Rotation of the spine in a leaned back position may not be suitable for certain disc-related back problems

Oblique lean backs with knee lifts

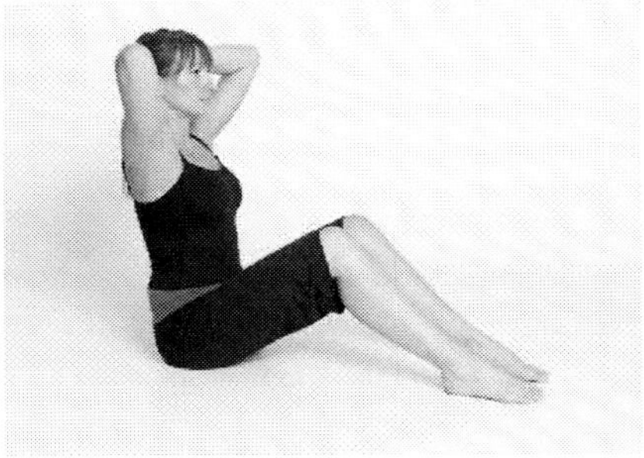

Aim

To work the oblique abdominals, whilst maintaining pelvic stability

Starting Position

Sit upright on the floor with the knees bent and the feet hip distance apart. Roll back slightly so that the pelvis is in a posterior tilt. The hands are clasped behind the head.

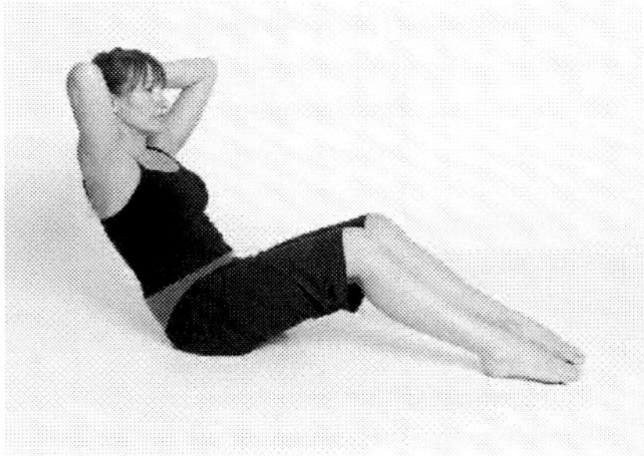

Action

Inhale - to prepare.

Exhale - engage the core abdominals and raise one foot off the floor until the knee is bent above the hip or wherever a neutral pelvis allows. Simultaneously oblique twist the torso to the right and lean back slightly, ensuring that the spine does not go into extension

Inhale - to prepare

Exhale - to lower the leg back down to the floor, keeping the abdominals engaged and return the body to the centre.

Repeat to the opposite side.

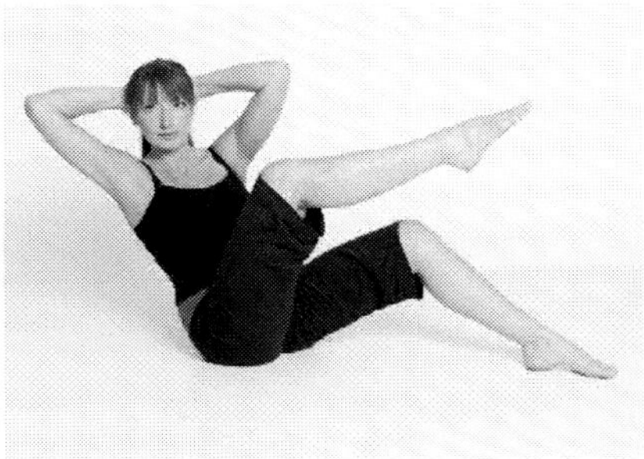

Target muscles

Core abdominals, hip flexors, obliques, scapula stabilisers

Watchpoints

- Keep the abdominals engaged throughout and prevent the lumbar spine going into extension
- Slide the shoulder blades down and apart so that the shoulders stay away from the ears and keep the neck long
- Try not to grip around the hip flexors
- Ensure the relationship between the elbows, shoulders and ears remains the same to avoid turning the head more than necessary or moving one elbow inwards
- Keep the elbows in front of the ears (i.e. within peripheral vision) and the fingers interlaced so that the hands act like a "hammock" cradling the head.

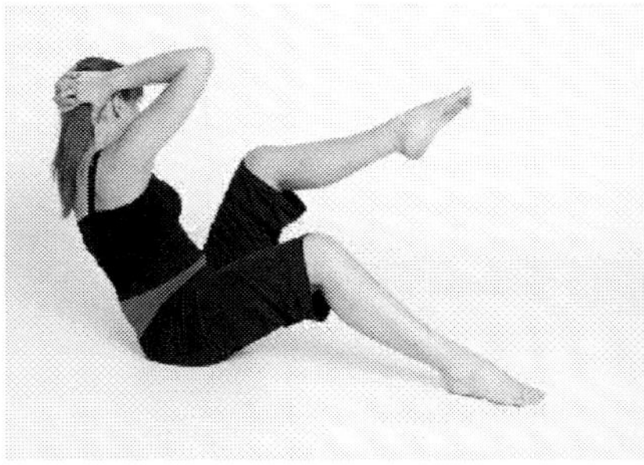

Contra-Indications

Twisting actions of the spine whilst in a leaned back position may be unsuitable for disc related back problems

Oblique curl ups

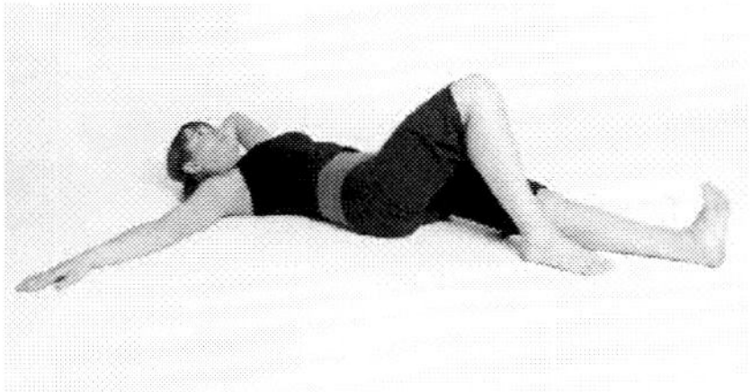
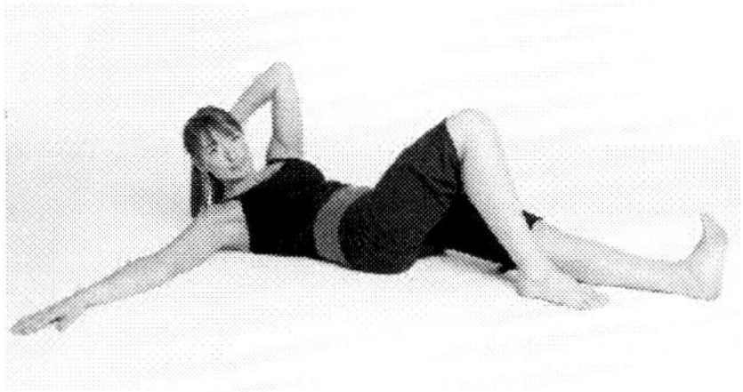
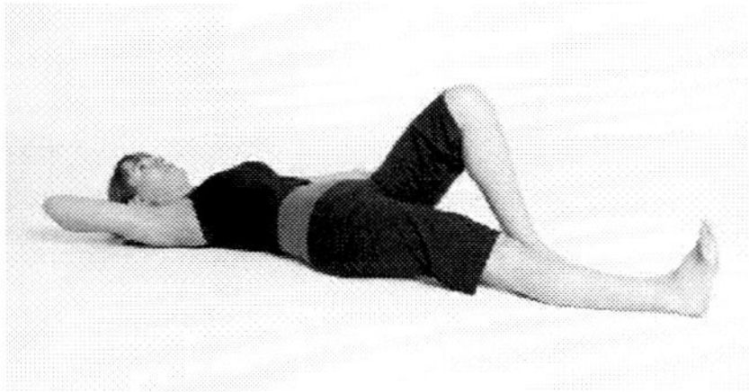
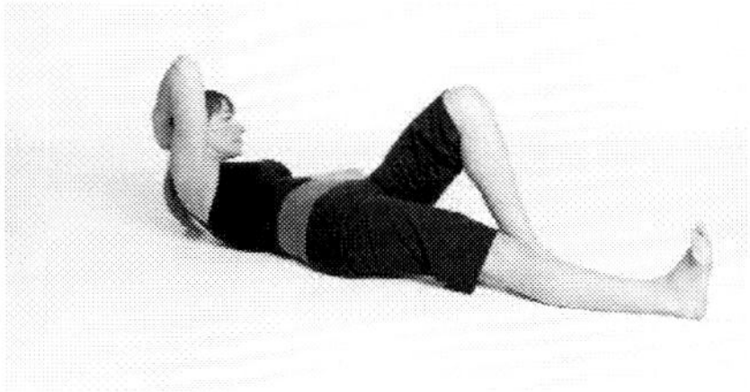

Aim

To work the abdominals, whilst maintaining pelvic stability

Starting Position

Lie supine with the knees bent and the legs together and the pelvis in neutral. Clasp the right hand behind the head and extend the right leg straight out along the floor. The left arm is outstretched at shoulder height along the floor, palm face down and the left knee remains bent.

Action

Inhale - to prepare.

Exhale - engage the core abdominals, tuck in the chin and raise the head and shoulders off the floor and oblique twist to the left in half curl-up position. The right elbow aims towards the left knee.

Inhale – to prepare

Exhale - hold that position in the air and perform ten little contractions, pulsing no more than one or two inches and increasing spinal flexion and abdominal contraction on each exhalation.

Repeat to the opposite side

Target muscles

Rectus abdominis, core abdominals, obliques, hip flexors

Watchpoints

- Keep the chin tucked in as if holding a small apple between the chin and the chest to avoid shortening the back of the neck
- Ensure the shoulders stay away from the ears
- Try not to turn the head more than necessary or move the elbow forwards during the twist
- Ensure that the opposite hip and buttock remain on the floor during the twist
- Do not over twist – aim for height and length
- Ensure the pelvis remains in a neutral position throughout

Variation One (Progression)

This exercise may be performed with a leg raise. Instead of the extended leg remaining on the floor, raise it a few inches off the floor (the closer to the floor, the harder) and the arm raises up towards the ceiling instead of being behind the head.

Contra-Indications

This exercise may be unsuitable for certain disc related back problems. A curl-up may not be suitable for those with osteoporosis of the spine

Criss Cross

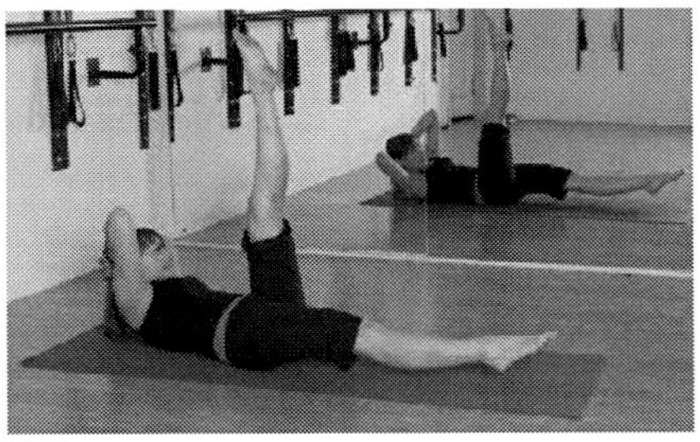

Aim

To work the abdominals, obliques abdominals and challenge co-ordination

Starting Position

Lie supine on the floor with the pelvis in neutral. Inhale to prepare and exhale to engage the core abdominals and raise one foot at a time of the floor until the legs are straight and directly above the hips. The legs are together and the toes are slightly pointed. The hands are clasped behind the head.

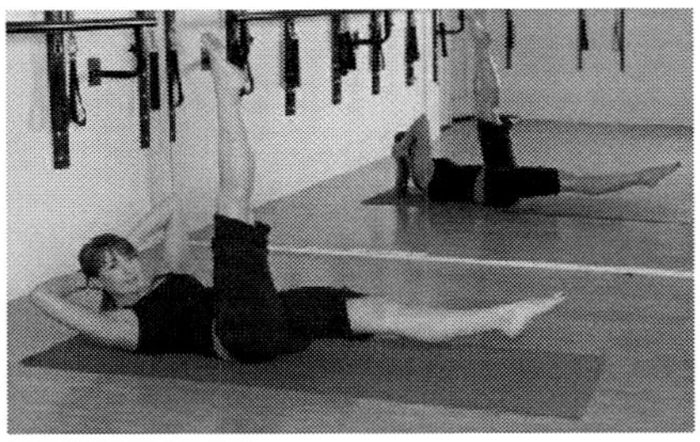

Action

Inhale - engage the core abdominals, and straighten the right leg away from the body. As the leg extends, twist the body to the left

Exhale – to hold the position and draw in the navel on the exhalation. The combination of drawing in the navel and exhaling will allow the body to lift a little higher

Inhale - to return the leg back to the starting position

Exhale – to repeat with the opposite leg, twisting to the other side

Target muscles

Rectus abdominis, core abdominals, hip flexors, obliques

Watchpoints

- Ensure that the pelvis remains in a neutral position throughout
- If the legs cannot straighten due to tight hamstrings or if the back starts to arch, then only straighten the legs as far as the body allows
- Ensure that the neck stays long and the shoulders stay away from the ears
- Try not to over twist otherwise one side of the pelvis will lift off the floor (i.e. the pelvis will tilt from east to west or vice versa depending upon which way the body is twisting)

Variation One (Adaptation)

This exercise may be performed with one leg bent and the other leg straight

Contra-Indications

Twisting of the spine may not be suitable for those with disc related back problems. Forward flexion of the spine may be unsuitable for osteoporosis.

Banana obliques

Aim

To work the oblique abdominals, whilst maintaining length in the waist

Starting Position

Lie on the left hand side of the body with the arms down by the sides, slightly in front of the body.

Action

Inhale - to prepare

Exhale - to engage the core abdominals and both legs off the floor. Simultaneously raise the head, shoulders and arms off the floor

Inhale - to return to the starting position.

Target Muscles

Oblique Abdominals, core abdominals, scapula stabilisers

Watchpoints

- Ensure the shoulders stay away from the ear and the gap between the ear and shoulder remains equal on both sides
- Keep the neck long and do not lead with the head as the body lifts. The cervical spine should be in alignment with the rest of the spine

Variation One (Adaptation)

Lifting two straight legs off the floor can put pressure on the spine and may prove uncomfortable. In this instance, only raise one leg in the air.

Variation Two (Progression)

Once both legs have lifted, roll the pelvis slightly backwards and twist the torso so that the shoulders are square to the ceiling and curl up higher. This is an advanced exercise and should only be attempted if lumbar flexion can be maintained.

Contra-Indications

This exercise may place stress on the neck. Take extra care when attempting this exercise for certain neck problems. If discomfort is felt in the spine when lifting two legs in the air, choose Variation One instead.

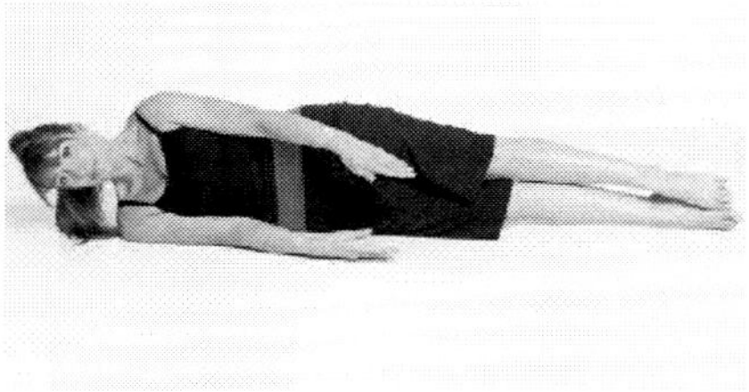

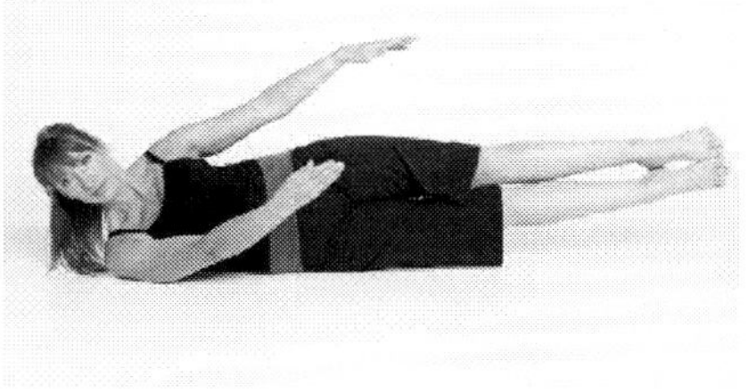

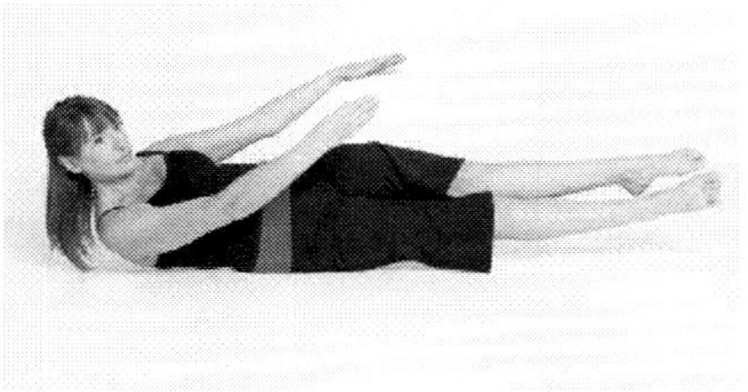

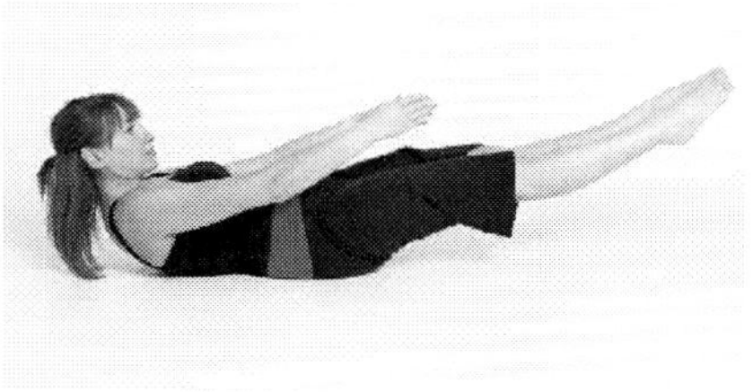

Variation Two

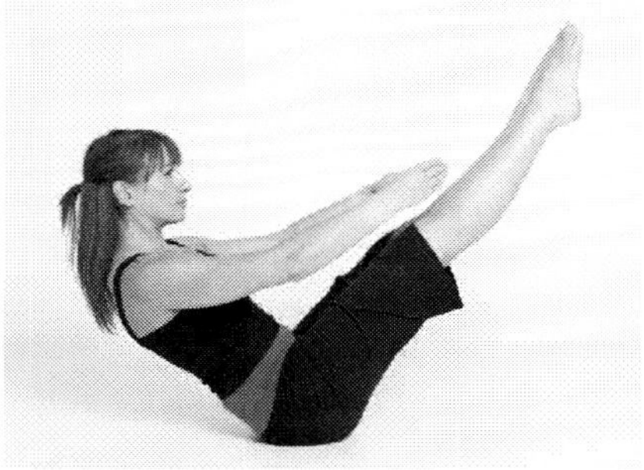

Variation Two

Pelvic Rocks

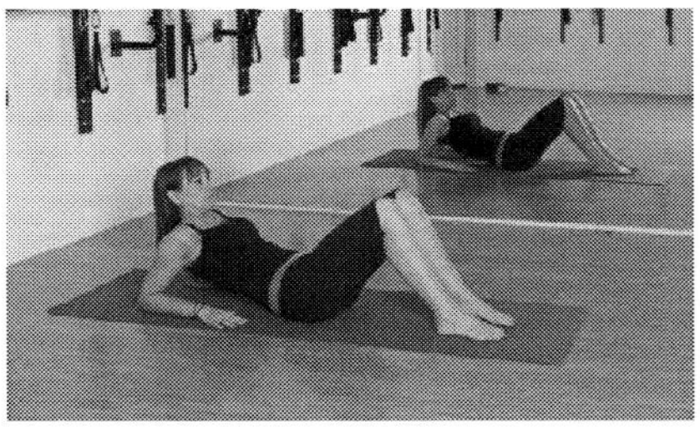

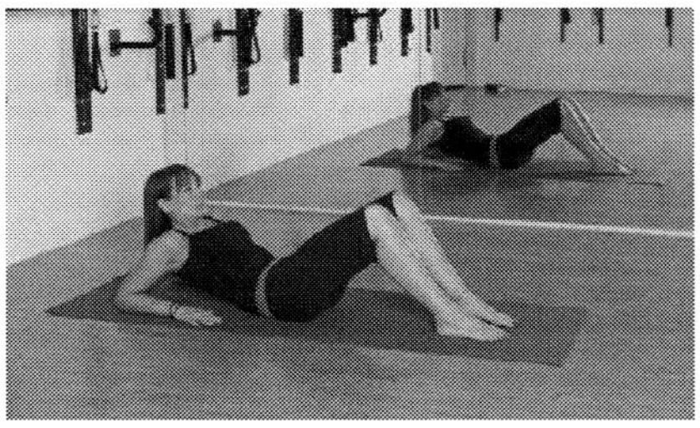

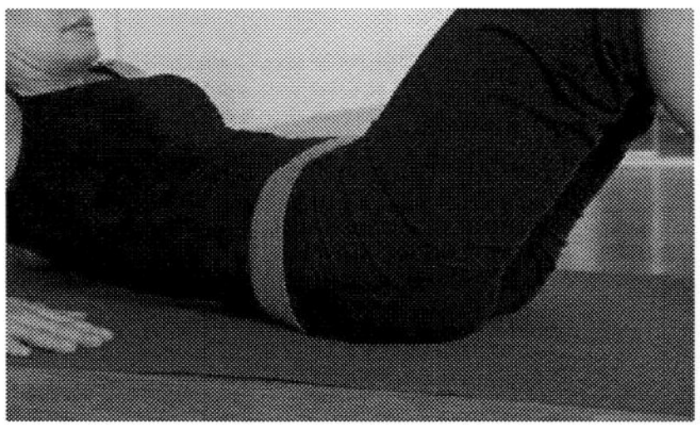

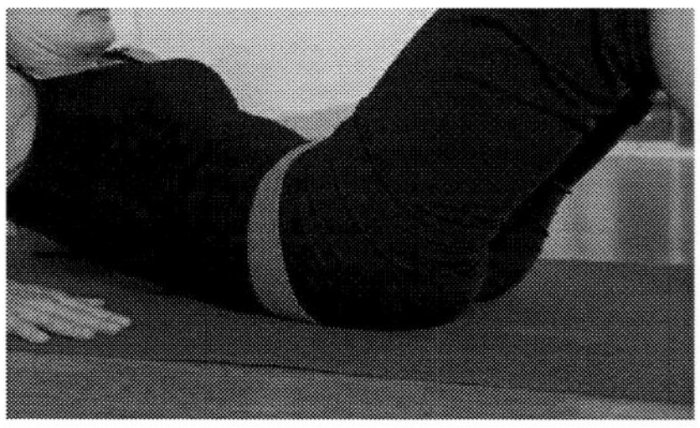

Aim

To work the abdominals in an imprinted position

Starting Position

Lie supine on the floor with the knees bent and feet hip distance apart. The pelvis is in neutral. Curl the head and shoulders off the floor and bend the elbows to prop the body up by resting on the elbows. The elbows should be behind the shoulders as far as flexibility allows.

Action

Inhale - to prepare

Exhale – to roll the pelvis back into a posterior tilt, whilst keeping the body stable and at the same height. The sacrum is aiming to press towards the floor. Hold for 5 seconds

Inhale – to return the pelvis back to neutral. Repeat these pelvic tilts up to 20 times.

Target Muscles

Core abdominals

Watchpoints

- Ensure that the neck stays long and shoulders stay away from the ears
- Do not collapse in between the shoulder blades – keep the collar bones open
- Keep the abdominals engaged throughout

Variation One (Adaptation)

This can be performed from an upright sitting positions. Roll back a few inches as for the previous Lean Backs exercise and perform the pelvic rocks from this position

Contra-Indications

This exercise may not be suitable for certain disc related back problems

Reverse Curl

Aim

To work m the abdominals and achieve segmental control of the spine and to stretch the back

Starting Position

Lie supine in the relaxation position with the knees bent. Inhale to prepare. As you exhale, engage the core abdominals and lift one leg up at a time until the legs are bent at 90 degrees above the hips. The arms are down by the side of the body.

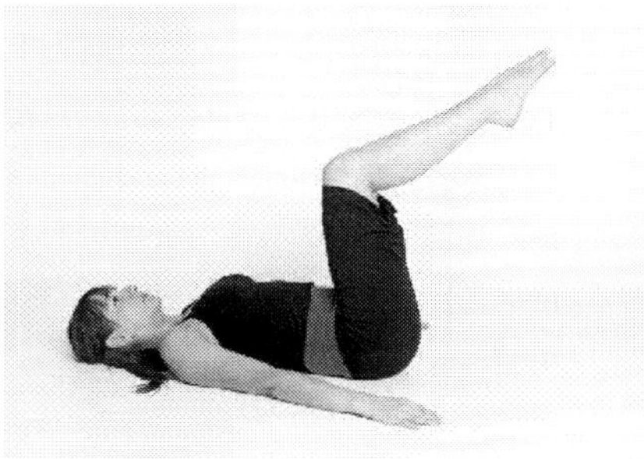

Action

Inhale - To prepare

Exhale - Engage the core abdominals and tilt the pelvis, lifting the tailbone, sacrum and lumbar spine off the floor

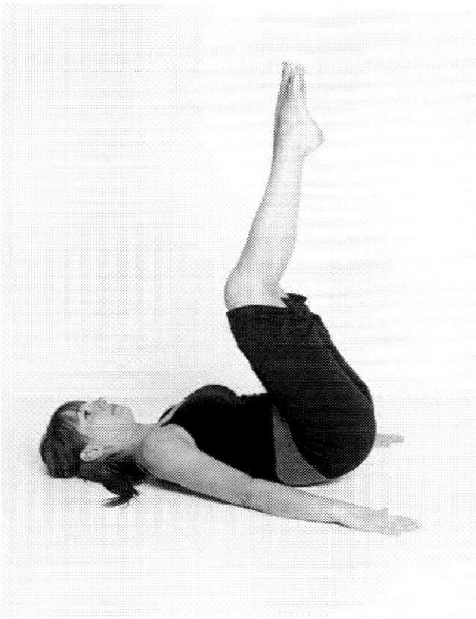

Inhale - To prepare

Exhale - Slowly reverse the movement to return back to the starting position. Use the hands to act as a brake by lightly pressing the palms into the floor.

Target Muscles

Core abdominals, hip flexors

Watchpoints

- As you come back to the starting position on the returning phase of the movement, ensure that the head stays on the floor
- Try to keep shoulders away from the ears
- Try to move sequentially, one vertebra at a time throughout the movement
- Ensure that the abdominals do not bulge. Keep them hollowed throughout
- Only lift as far as the lumbar spine and no higher

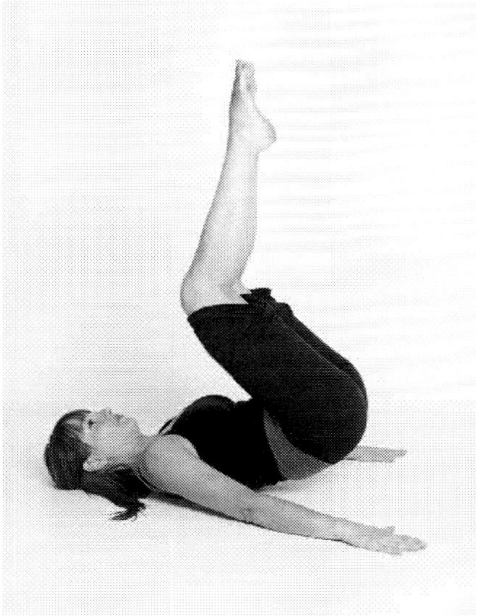

Contra-Indications

This exercise may be unsuitable for certain disc related back problems and osteoporosis

Toe Taps

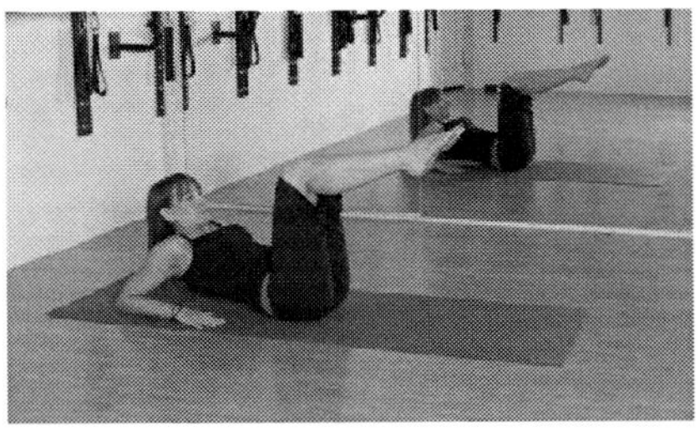

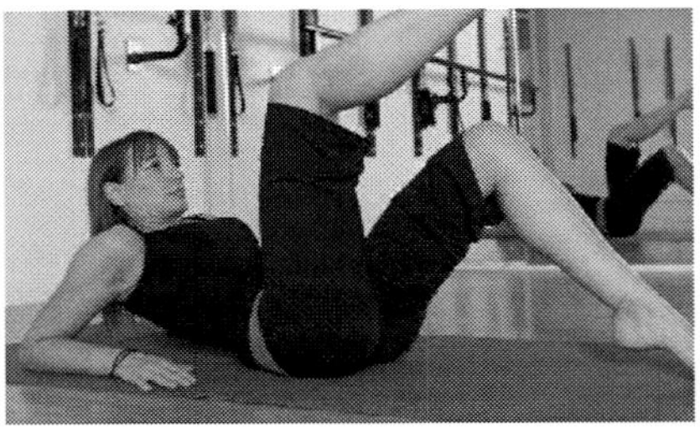

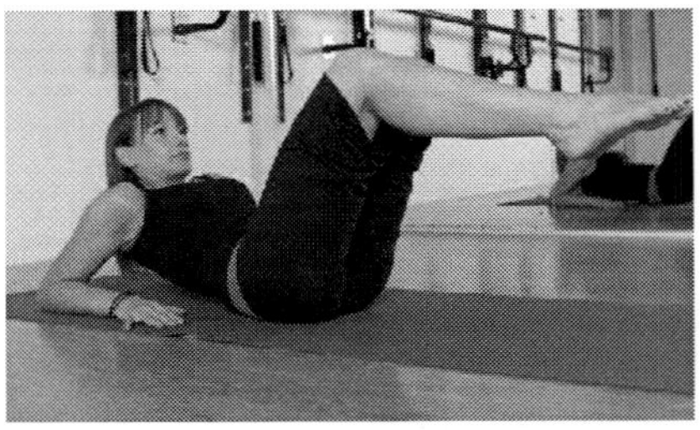

Variation Four

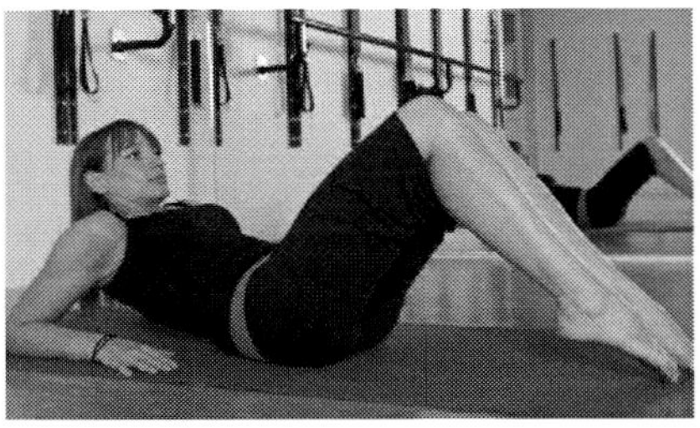

Variation Four

Aim

To work the abdominals whilst maintaining pelvic stability

Starting Position

Lie supine on the floor with the knees bent and feet hip distance apart. The pelvis is in neutral. Curl the head and shoulders off the floor and bend the elbows to prop the body up by resting on the elbows. The elbows should be behind the shoulders as far as flexibility allows. Engage the core abdominals and raise one foot at a time off the floor until the knees are bent at around 90 degrees above the hips. Imprint the spine into the floor by bringing the pelvis into a posterior tilt and increasing lumbar flexion.

Action

Inhale - To prepare

Exhale - To lower the first leg down towards the floor. Ideally the big toe will tap the floor. Hold for 5 seconds

Inhale - To bring the leg back up above the hip again

Exhale - To lower the opposite leg to the floor and hold for 5 seconds

Inhale - To bring the leg back up above the hip again

Target muscles

Rectus abdominis, core abdominals, hip flexors

Watchpoints

- Ensure that the pelvis remains in a stable imprinted position throughout
- Ensure that the neck stays long and shoulders stay away from the ears
- Do not collapse in between the shoulder blades – keep the collar bones open
- Keep the abdominals engaged throughout

Variation One (Adaptation)

This exercise may be done lying supine in the relaxation position with the head on the floor if being propped up on the elbows is uncomfortable

Variation Two (Adaptation)

Instead of lifting both legs, this exercise may be made easier if only one leg lifts (single knee raises). Inhale to prepare. As you exhale, engage the core abdominals and raise one foot off the floor until the knee is bent at around 90 degrees above the hip. Inhale to prepare. As you exhale, engage the core abdominals and lower the leg back down to the floor again. Repeat with the opposite leg.

Variation Three (Progression)

This exercise may be done in a half curl up position without being propped up on the elbows. Place both hands behind the knees and release one hand as the same leg lowers down. More advanced would be to have the arms in the air, whilst performing the toe taps in a half curled position.

Variation Four (Progression)

Double toe taps. Inhale to prepare and exhale to lower both legs back down to the floor as far as a stable pelvis allows. Inhale to return the legs back above the hips again.

Scissors

Aim

To use the core abdominals to secure a neutral pelvis whilst moving the legs

Starting Position

Lie supine in the relaxation position with the knees bent. Inhale to prepare. As you exhale, engage the core abdominals and lift one leg up at a time until the legs are directly above the hips at 90 degrees. Straighten the legs as much as possible ensuring that the knees stay directly above the hips. For tight hamstrings, the knees may be bent as necessary. Curl the head and shoulders off the floor and stretch the arms along the floor, palms face down on the floor.

Action

Inhale - to prepare.

Exhale - engage the core abdominals and push the right leg away from the chest as far as a neutral pelvis can be maintained.

Inhale - to return to the starting position, keeping abdominals hollowed.

Repeat with the opposite leg.

Target Muscles

Core abdominals, hamstrings, hip flexors

Watchpoints

- Ensure the neck stays long and shoulders are away from the ears
- Keep the abdominals hollowed and only move the legs as far as a neutral pelvis can be maintained
- For tight hamstrings or to make the exercise easier, the knees may stay as bent as necessary

Variation One (Adaptation)

This exercise may be performed with the head and shoulders on the floor if discomfort in the neck is felt

Variation Two (Progression)

This exercise may be performed with the arms gently holding behind the thighs

Variation Three (Progression)

This exercise may be performed with the arms in the air above the shoulders

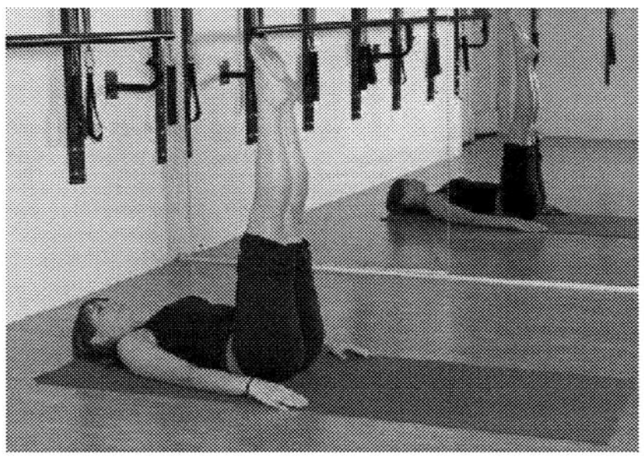

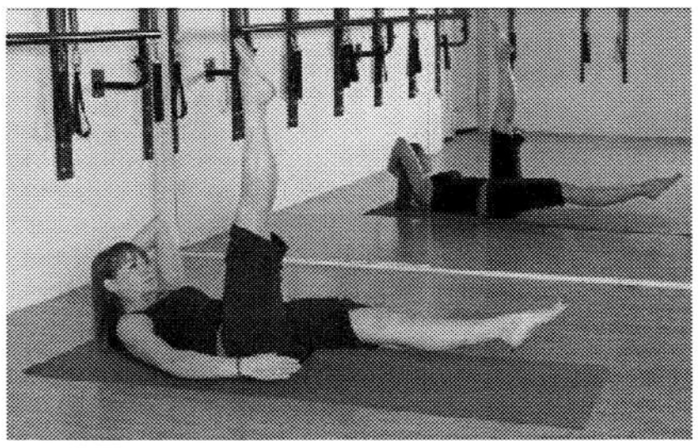

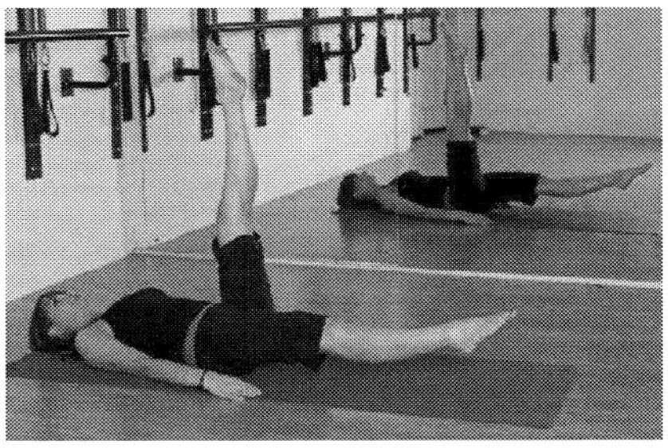

Variation One

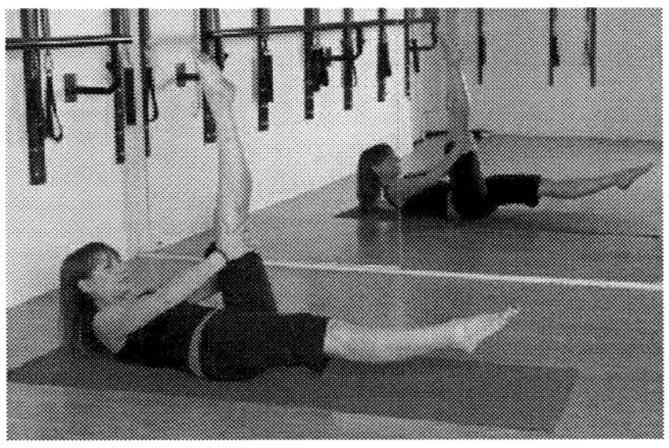

Variation Two

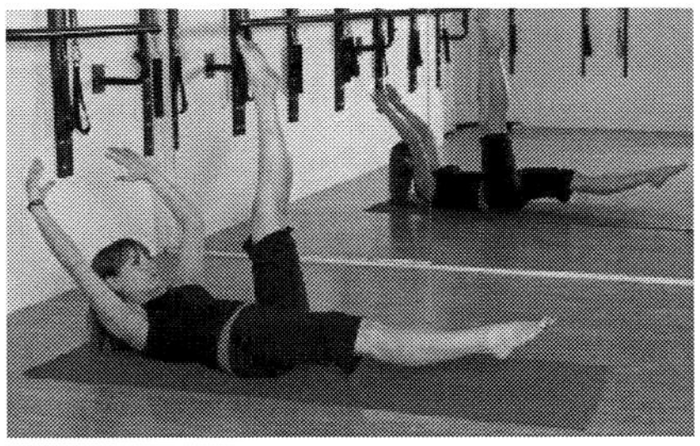

Variation Three

Diamond Leg Lowers

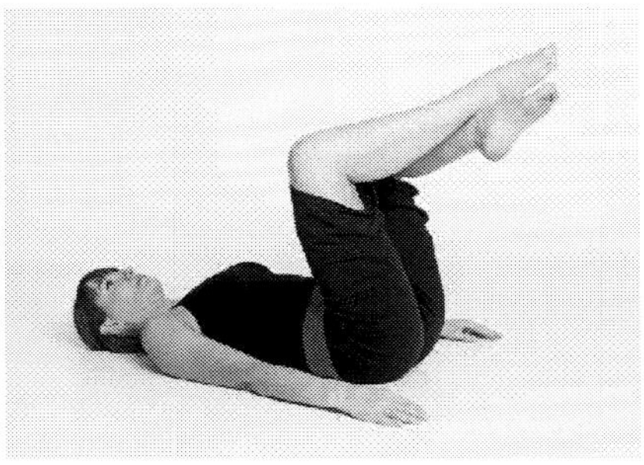

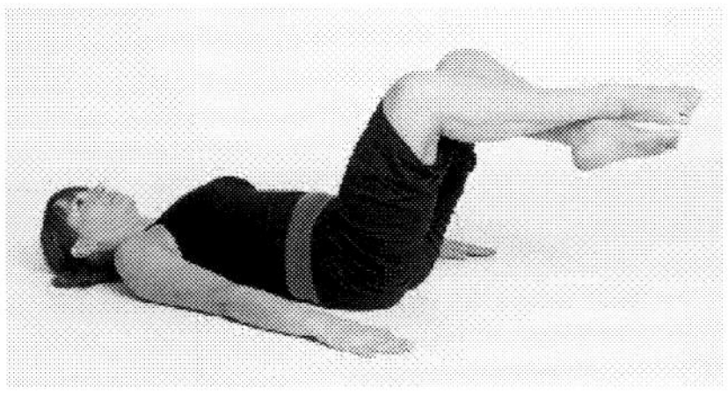

Aim

To work the abdominals, whilst maintaining pelvic stability

Starting Position

Lie supine on the floor with the pelvis in neutral. The arms are down by the sides of the body on the floor. Inhale to prepare and exhale to engage the core abdominals and raise one foot at a time of the floor until the knees are bent at around 90 degrees above the hips. Open out the knees to shoulder width apart and criss cross one ankle over the other and the toes are slightly pointed.

Action

Inhale - to prepare

Exhale - engage the core abdominals, and lower the thighs away from the body so that the feet come towards the floor as far as a neutral pelvis can be maintained. The angle at the knee remains at around 90 degrees throughout

Inhale - as the legs return back in towards the body.

Target muscles

Core abdominals, hip flexors

Watchpoints

- Ensure that the pelvis remains in a neutral position throughout
- Ensure that the neck stays long and the shoulders stay away from the ears
- Only move the leg as far as a neutral pelvis can be maintained
- Keep the knees at a 90 degree angle throughout

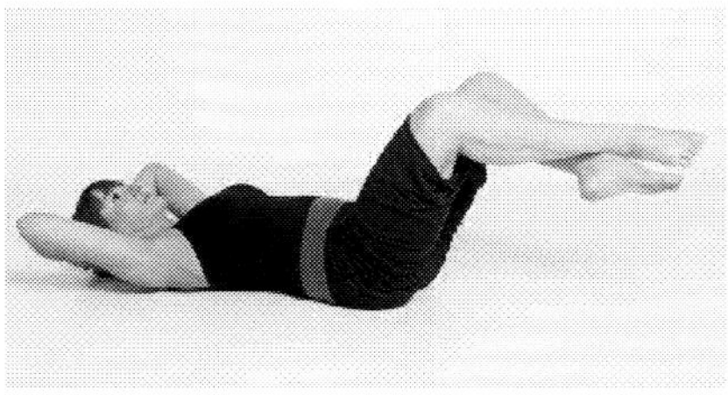

Variation Two

Variation One (Adaptation)

Only push one leg away from the body if the weight of two legs is too much

Variation Two (Progression)

The arms may be in the air, directly above the shoulders (easier), or outstretched behind the head (harder).

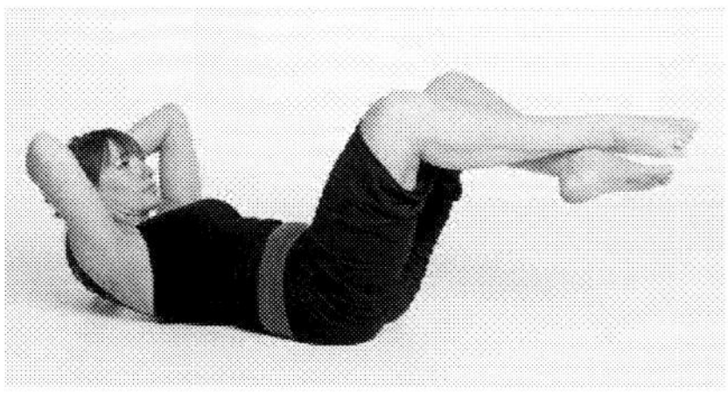

Variation Four

Variation Three (Progression)

Once the legs have been pushed away, the feet may then push forwards (thereby straightening the legs) as far as a stable pelvis allows

Variation Four (Progression)

An abdominal curl up may be added as the legs push away

Double leg press

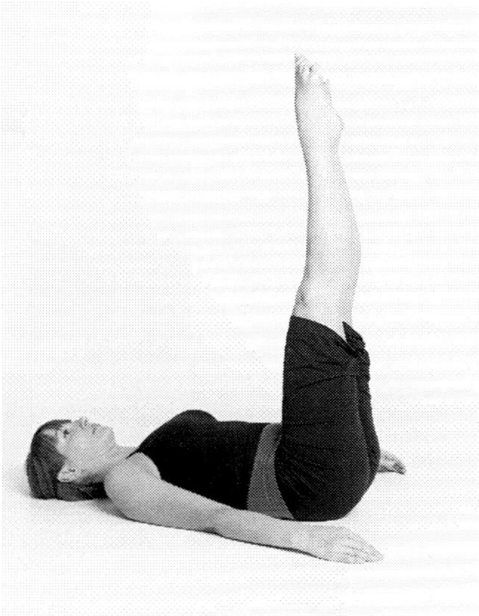

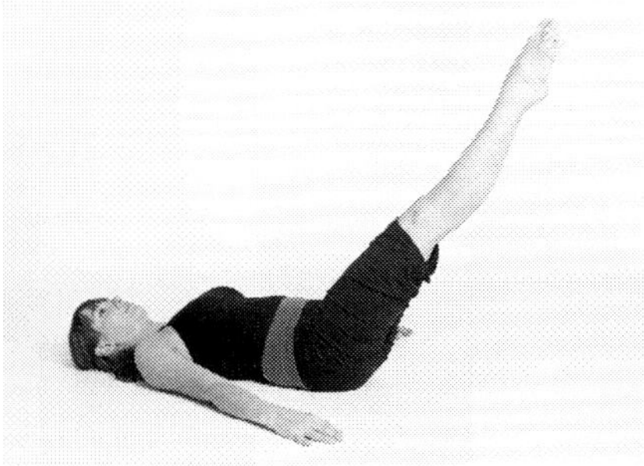

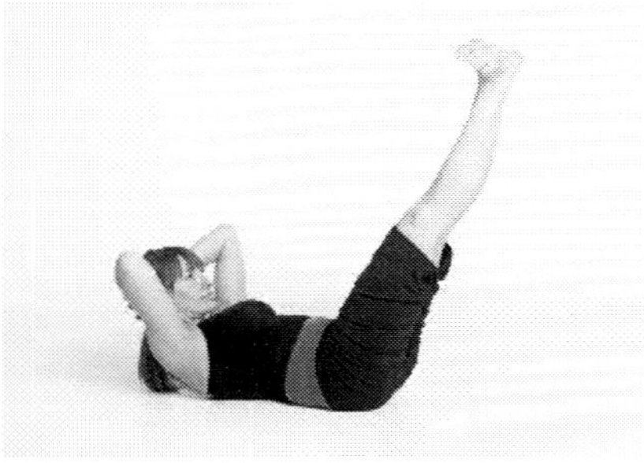

Variation Two

Aim

To work the abdominals whilst maintaining a neutral pelvis

Starting Position

Lie supine in the relaxation position with knees bent and the feet hip width apart. Inhale to prepare. As you exhale, engage the core abdominals and lift one leg up at a time until the legs are bent at 90 degrees above the hips. Straighten the legs as much as possible ensuring that the knees stay directly above the hips. For tight hamstrings, the knees may be bent. The arms are down by the sides of the body.

Action

Inhale - To prepare

Exhale - Engage the core abdominals and push the legs away from the chest and towards the floor as far as a neutral pelvis can be maintained

Inhale - To return to the starting position.

Target Muscles

Core abdominals, hip flexors

Watchpoints

- Ensure neck stays long and shoulders are away from the ears
- Keep abdominals hollowed and only move the legs as far as a neutral pelvis can be maintained

Variation One (Adaptation)

To make the exercise easier, the knees may stay as bent as is necessary

Variation Two (Progression)

This exercise may be performed with the head off floor throughout and the hands clasped behind the head.

Double Leg Stretch

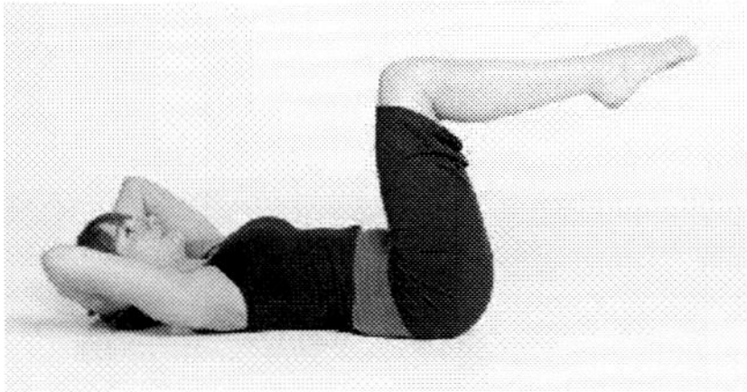

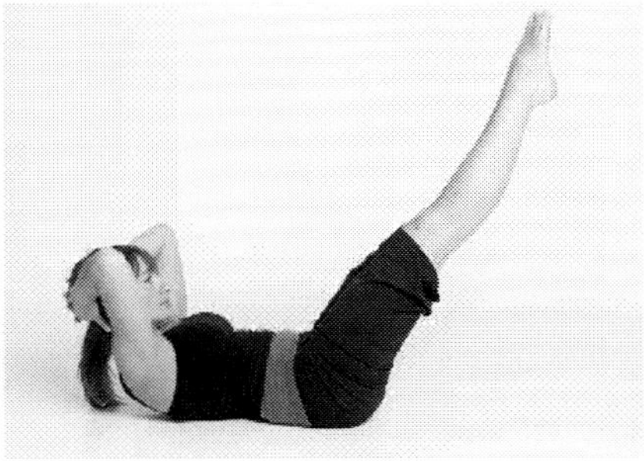

Aim

To work the deep and superficial abdominals whilst maintaining stability in the pelvis

Starting Position

Lie supine in the relaxation position with knees bent. Inhale to prepare. As you exhale, engage the core abdominals and lift one leg up at a time until the legs are bent at 90 degrees above the hips. Clasp the hands behind the head

Action

Inhale - To prepare

Exhale - To engage the core abdominals and extend the legs as straight as possible and simultaneously curl the head and shoulders off the floor

Inhale - To bend the knees back to 90 degrees and return the torso back to the floor. The closer/lower the legs are to the floor, the more challenging the exercise.

Target Muscles

Core Abdominals

Watchpoints

- Keep abdominals hollowed and only move the legs as far as a neutral pelvis can be maintained
- Keep the chin tucked in as if holding a small apple between the chin and the chest to avoid shortening the back of the neck
- Slide the shoulder blades down and apart so that the shoulders stay away from the ears
- Keep the elbows in front of the ears (i.e. within peripheral vision) and the fingers interlaced so that the hands act like a "hammock" cradling the head. This way, the hands take the weight of the head and not the neck and so this avoids neck strain.

Contra-Indications

A curled up position may not be suitable for certain disc-related back problems or osteoporosis

Floorwork Pliés

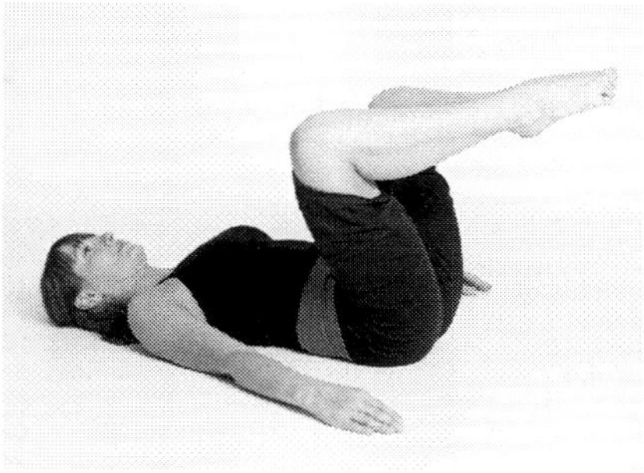

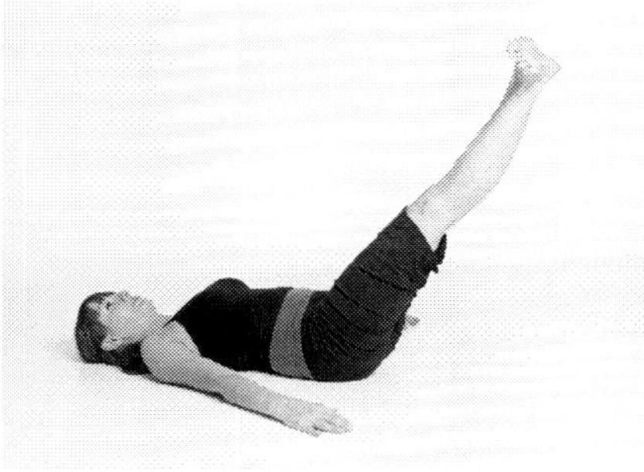

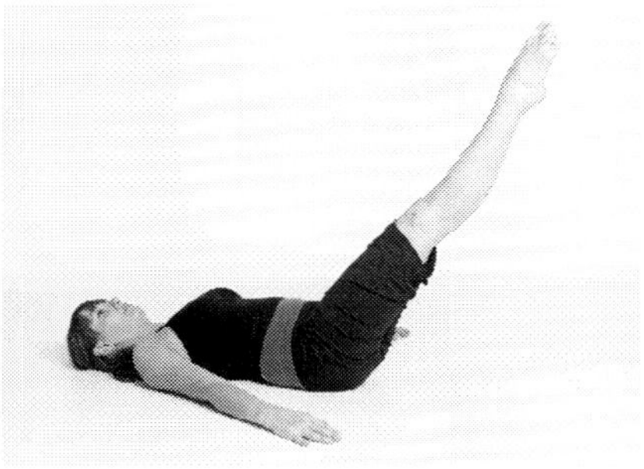

Aim

To work the abdominals and practice working in external rotation

Starting Position

Lie supine on the floor with the pelvis in neutral. The arms are down by the sides of the body on the floor. Inhale to prepare and exhale to engage the core abdominals and raise one foot at a time of the floor until the knees are bent at around 90 degrees above the hips. Turn out the legs in the hip sockets so that the knees are slightly wider than the hips. The feet are pointed and the heels are level with the knees.

Action

Inhale - to prepare

Exhale - engage the core abdominals, and straighten the legs as much as possible, pointing the toes and maintaining the turned out position. The legs aim to straighten at an angle of between 30-80 degrees. The closer the legs are to the floor, the more challenging the exercise.

Inhale – to flex the feet

Exhale – to point the toes

Inhale – to bend the knees and return to the starting position

Target muscles

Rectus abdominis, core abdominals, hip flexors, adductors, gluteals, external leg rotators, gastrocnemus

Watchpoints

- Ensure that the pelvis remains in a neutral position throughout
- If the legs cannot straighten due to tight hamstrings or if the back starts to arch, then only straighten the legs as far as the body allows
- Ensure that the neck stays long and the shoulders stay away from the ears

Variation One (Adaptation)

This exercise may be done in parallel if the turned out position is unsuitable

Contra-Indications

This exercise may be unsuitable for those with sciatica since the turned out position may aggravate this condition. Choose variation one instead.

Frogs

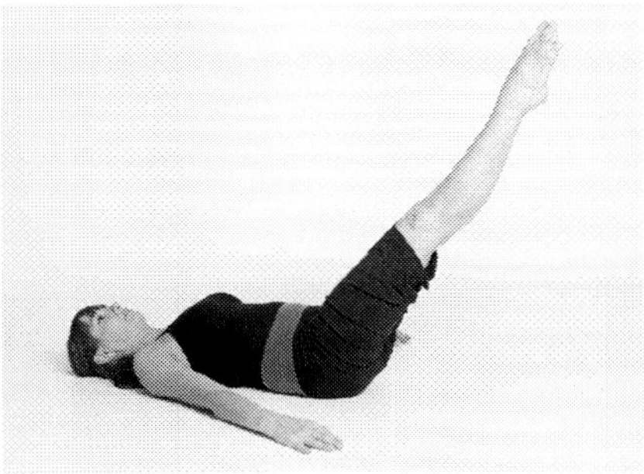

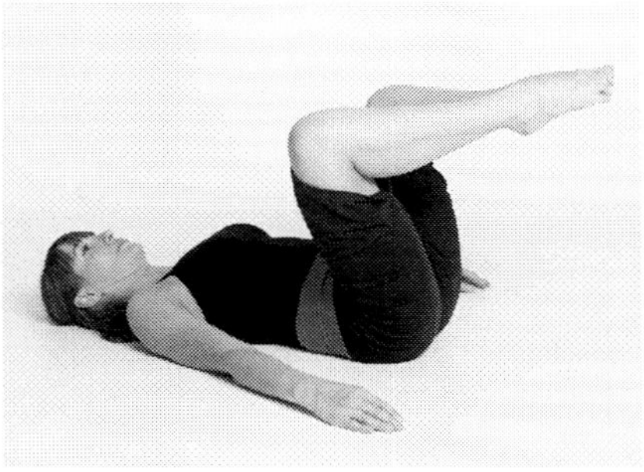

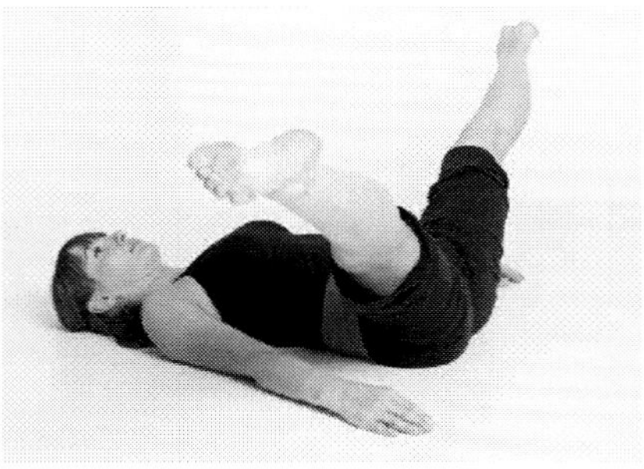

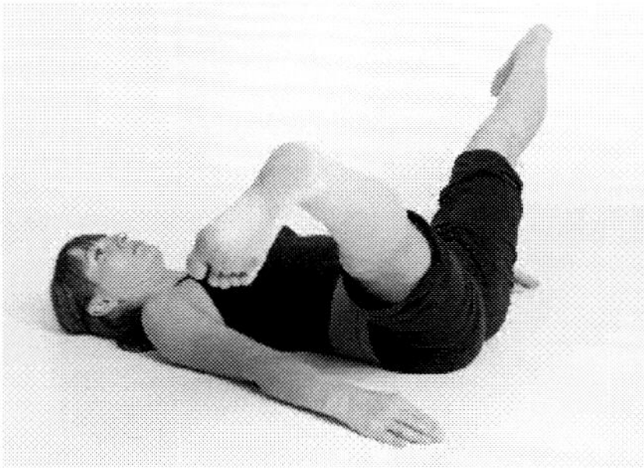

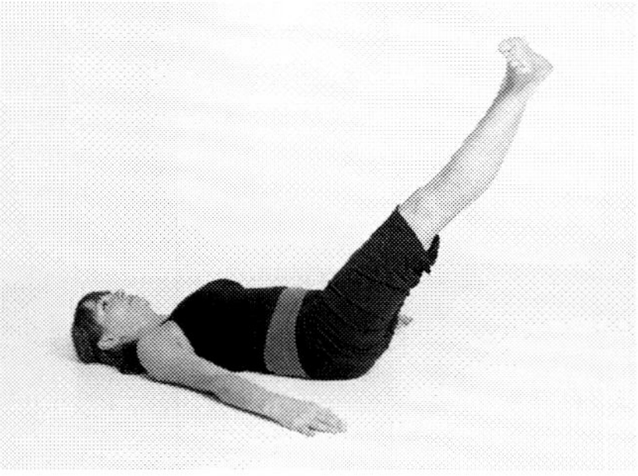

Aim

To strengthen the abdominals, whilst working in turn out and to maintain pelvic stability

Starting Position

Lie supine in the relaxation position with knees bent and the feet hip width apart. Inhale to prepare. As you exhale, engage the core abdominals and lift one leg up at a time until the legs are bent at 90 degrees above the hips. Extend the legs away from the body to around 45 degrees and externally rotate them in the hip sockets. The feet are pointed.

Action

Inhale – To engage the powerhouse and bend the knees in towards the chest as far as a neutral pelvis allows. The knees are around shoulder width apart with the toes pointed together

Exhale – To open out the legs to the side, maintaining the same position of the knee in space

Inhale – To flex the feet

Exhale – To push the legs away to 45 degrees and adduct them together to return to the starting position

Reverse the direction.

Start with the legs extended at 45 degrees. Inhale to open out the legs to the side. Exhale flex the feet. Inhale to bend the knees and bring the heels together, keeping the knees around shoulder width apart. Exhale to extend the legs, pushing them away and adducting them together to around 45 degrees

Target Muscles

Hamstrings, hip flexors, core abdominals, gluteals, adductors, quadriceps, lateral rotators

Watchpoints

- Ensure good use of the core abdominals throughout to prevent any unwanted movement of the pelvis. Limit the range of movement to where a neutral pelvis can be maintained.
- Ensure good oblique engagement to prevent the ribs flaring as the legs push away
- Ensure that both legs are working equally
- Keep the collar bones open, the neck long and the shoulders relaxed
- Get a sense of opposition and length as the legs push away
- A smooth flow and even speed is aimed for
- Keep the range of movement small initially. Once competent, the legs may open wider

Variation One

The feet may be flexed throughout or pointed throughout

Contra-Indications

turned out position may be unsuitable for sciatica.

Leg circles apart

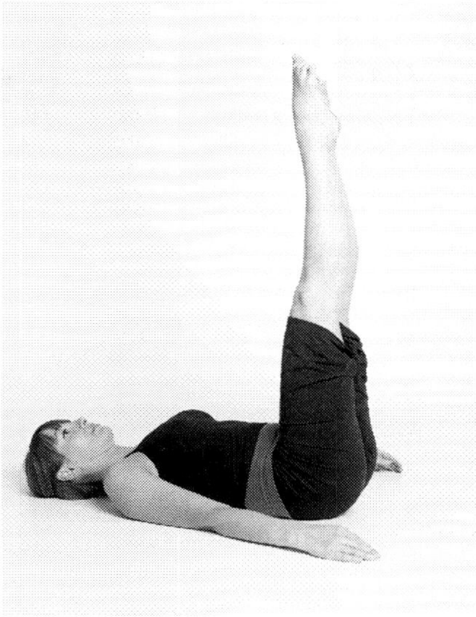

Aim

This exercise works the core abdominals and mobilises the hip joints

Starting Position

Lie supine in the relaxation position with knees bent and the feet hip width apart. Inhale to prepare. As you exhale, engage the core abdominals and lift one leg up at a time until the legs are bent at 90 degrees above the hips. Straighten the legs as much as possible ensuring that the knees stay directly above the hips. For tight hamstrings, the knees may be bent. Externally rotate the legs out in the hip socket. The arms are down by the side of the body.

Action

Inhale – To prepare

Exhale – To open out the legs to the side just wider than shoulder width apart. Continue exhaling to push the legs away from the chest to around 45 degrees. The legs remain at around 45 degrees throughout. Aim to draw small circles with the legs but they remain apart.

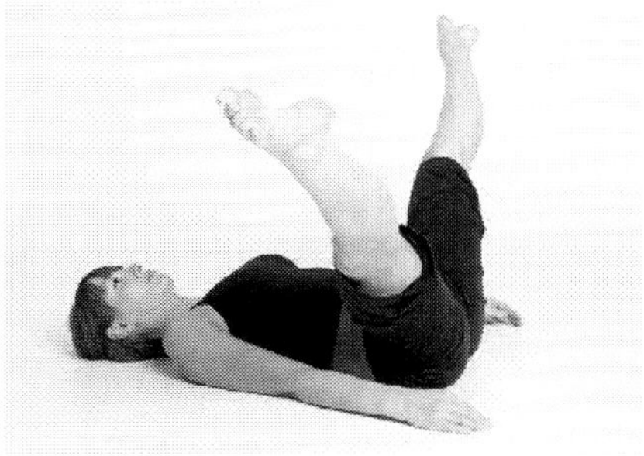

The direction should be reversed after a few repetitions. Whichever direction the legs travel, the breathing is always to exhale as the legs move away from the body and inhale to bring them towards the chest

Target Muscles

Hip flexors, core abdominals, gluteals, adductors, external rotators

Watchpoints

- Keep abdominals hollowed and only move the legs as far as a neutral pelvis can be maintained
- Keep the chin tucked in as if holding a small apple between the chin and the chest to avoid shortening the back of the neck
- Slide the shoulder blades down and apart so that the shoulders stay away from the ears

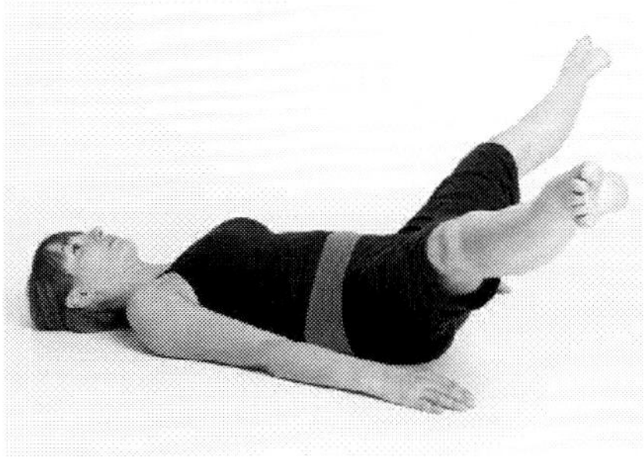

Variation One (Adaptation)

The legs may be lower or higher than 45 degrees, depending upon competency. The circles can be small initially with a greater range of movement when proficient.

Variation Two (Adaptation)

This may be done in a parallel position

Contra-Indications

A turned out position may be unsuitable for sciatica.

Half curls up with leg abduction

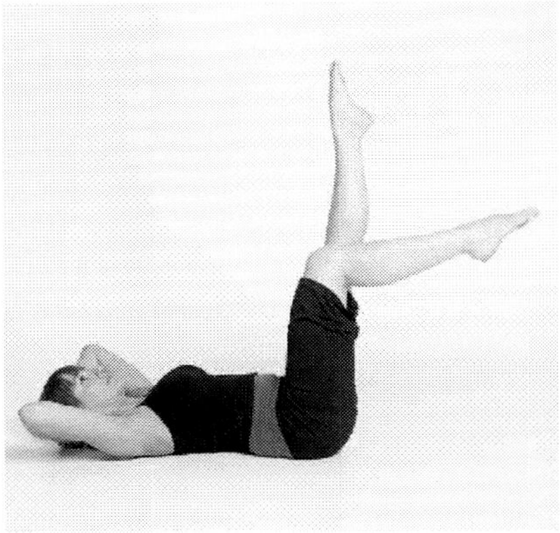

Aim

To work the oblique and core abdominals, whilst maintaining pelvic stability

Starting Position

Lie in the relaxation position. Inhale to prepare. Exhale, engage the core abdominals and raise one leg off the floor at a time until the knees are bent at 90 degrees above the hips. Keeping the knees together, straighten the left leg up to the ceiling, whilst the right leg stays bent at 90 degrees. Clasp the hands behind the head with the fingers interlaced and the elbows forward, within the peripheral vision.

Action

Inhale - to prepare

Exhale - to curl the head and upper back off the floor. Simultaneously open the right knee out to the right side as far as a neutral pelvis allows. The left leg stays straight with the foot being directly above the left hip

Inhale - to close the leg and return the head back down to the floor. Repeat with the opposite leg.

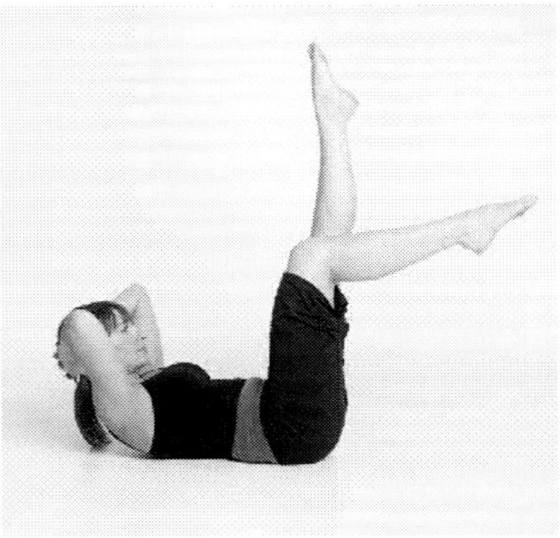

Target muscles

Core abdominals, rectus abdominis, obliques, abductors

Watchpoints

- Keep the chin tucked in as if holding a small apple between the chin and the chest to avoid shortening the back of the neck
- Slide the shoulder blades down and apart so that the shoulders stay away from the ears
- Keep the elbows in front of the ears (i.e. within peripheral vision) and the fingers interlaced so that the hands act like a "hammock" cradling the head. This way, the hands take the weight of the head and not the neck and so this avoids neck strain.
- Imagine a piece of sellotape on the trunk so that as you lift, try to keep the sellotape long and prevent it from squashing together (i.e. do not "crunch" – keep the trunk long)
- Only curl up as high as a neutral pelvis allows
- Keep the hipbones level. Only move the bent leg out to the side as far as a neutral pelvis allows (i.e. ensure the pelvis does not move east to west or vice versa)
- Ensure the straight leg does not move out in the opposite direction to the bent leg in order to compensate to keep the pelvis level. The foot should be in alignment with the hip.

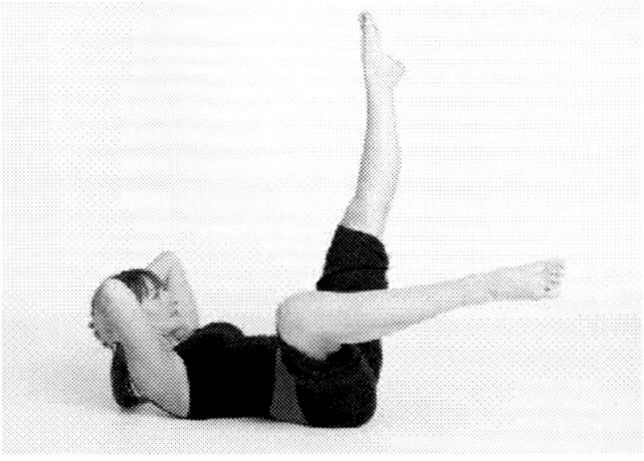

Variation One (Adaptation)

This exercise can be performed with the head on the floor. The curl up is left out and only the leg movement is performed for the core abdominals.

Variation Two (Progression)

To make this exercise more challenging, move the legs further away from the chest as the body curls-up. The further away the legs, the more difficult the exercise.

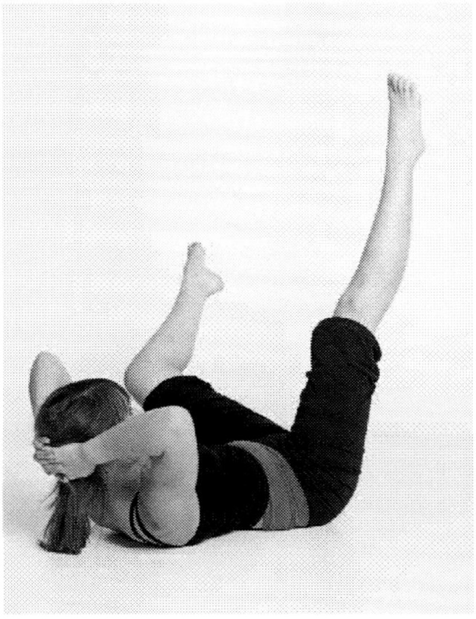

Contra-Indications

A curl-up may not be suitable for those with osteoporosis of the spine

Take care for those with neck problems, as this exercise may prove unsuitable

Half curl up with leg raise

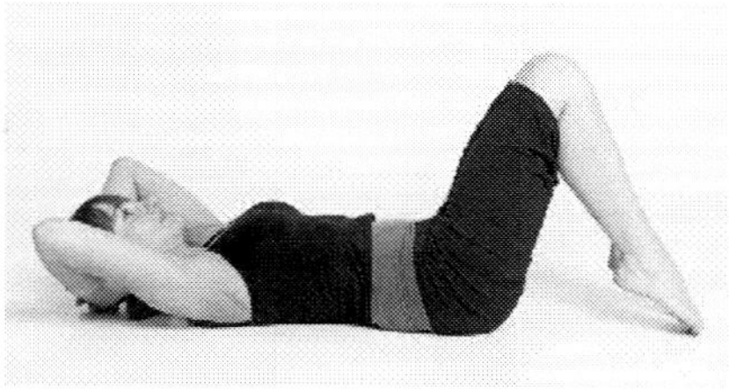
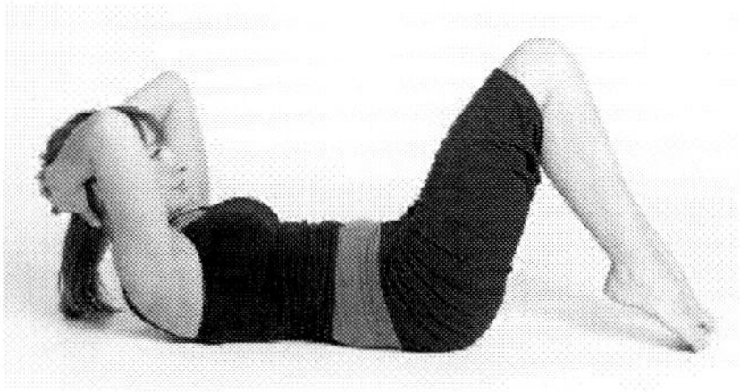
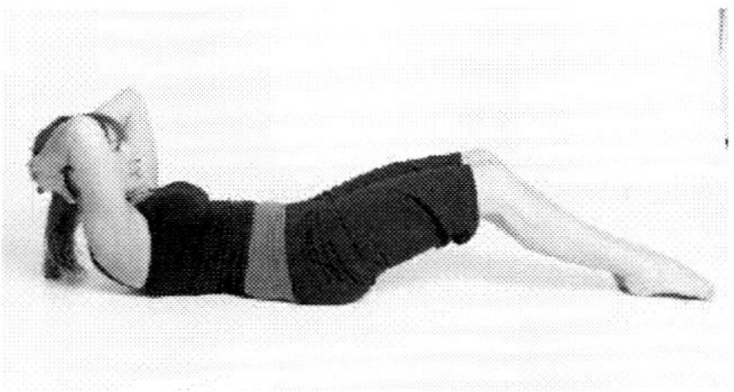
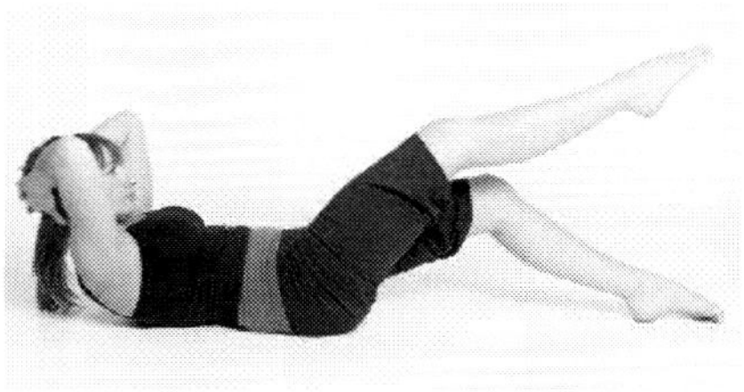
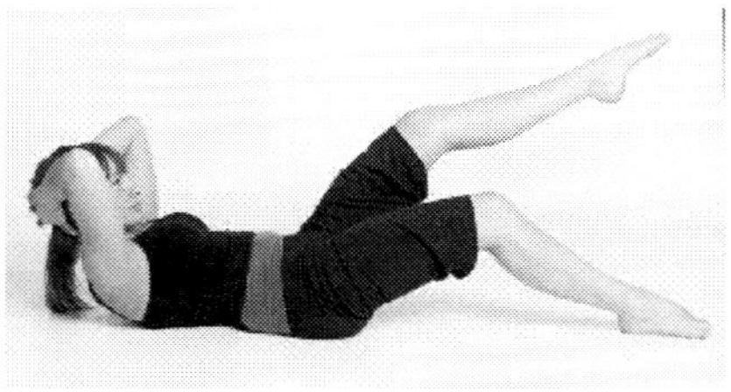

Aim

To work the abdominals, whilst maintaining pelvic stability

Starting Position

Lie supine with the knees bent and the legs together. The hands are clasped behind the head. Lift the heels off the floor and bring the feet to demi pointe.

Action

Inhale - to prepare.

Exhale - engage the core abdominals, tuck in the chin and raise the head and shoulders off the floor into a half curl-up position.

Inhale - and hold that position in the air

Exhale - to slide the legs away, extending the legs as straight as a stable spine will allow. (The further away the legs, the harder it is to maintain a stable pelvis)

Inhale - to prepare

Exhale - to raise the right leg off the floor without arching the back. Ensure you don't push the weight of the left leg into the floor

Inhale - as the right leg is placed back down on the floor

Repeat with the left leg (the higher the leg lifts, the less challenging the exercise and therefore the easier it is to maintain a neutral spine).

Exhale - to bend the knees back to return the feet and legs back to the start position and curl the upper body higher into flexion.

Inhale - to lower the torso back down.

Target muscles

Rectus abdominis, core abdominals, hip flexors

Watchpoints

- Keep the chin tucked in as if holding a small apple between the chin and the chest to avoid shortening the back of the neck
- Ensure the shoulders stay away from the ears
- Watch the back does not arch. Only straighten the legs if a stable spine can be maintained
- Only raise the leg if a stable pelvis can be maintained. If unstable, try lifting the straight leg higher towards the ceiling as this will make it easier

Variation One (Adaptation)

This exercise may be performed without the leg raise

Contra-Indications

For excessive lordosis, this position may prove too uncomfortable. This may also be unsuitable for certain disc related back problems. A curl-up may not be suitable for those with osteoporosis of the spine

Full curl ups

Aim

To work the abdominals whilst achieving segmental control of the spine

Starting Position

Lie supine with the legs adducted and outstretched on the floor and the arms down by the sides of the body.

Action

Inhale - To prepare

Exhale - To engage the core abdominals, tuck in the chin and raise the arms in the air. Slowly lift the head and torso off the floor, one vertebra at a time until fully sitting upright

Inhale – To fold forward into a hamstring stretch

Exhale - To sit upright and slowly return to the starting position, one vertebra at a time.

Target Muscles

Rectus abdominis, transverses abdominis

Watchpoints

- Keep the chin tucked in as if holding a small apple between the chin and the chest to avoid the tendency to shorten the back of the neck
- Ensure the shoulders stay away from the ears
- Try not to grip around the hip flexors
- Try to move segmentally through each vertebra, one at a time

Variation One (Adaptation)

Half curl ups. Clasp the hands behind the head and raise the head and shoulders off the floor. Perform to full range (i.e. from floor until shoulder blades are off the floor) or end range pulses.

Variation Two (Progression)

This exercise can be performed with knees bent

Contra-Indications

This exercise may not be suitable for certain disc-related back problems or osteoporosis

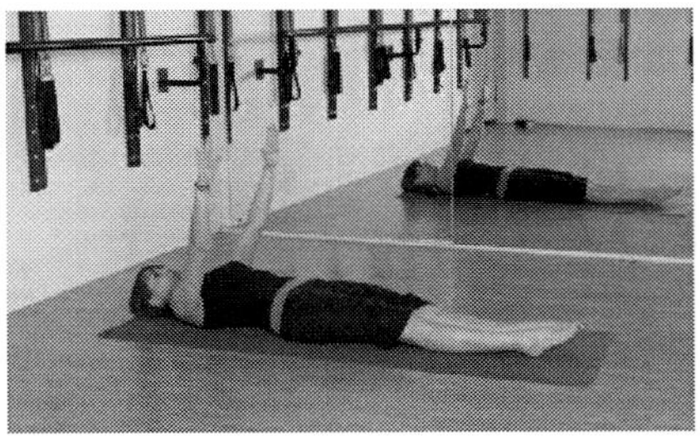

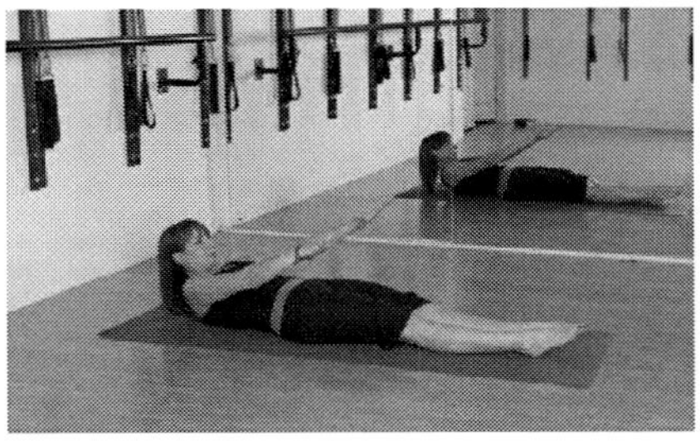

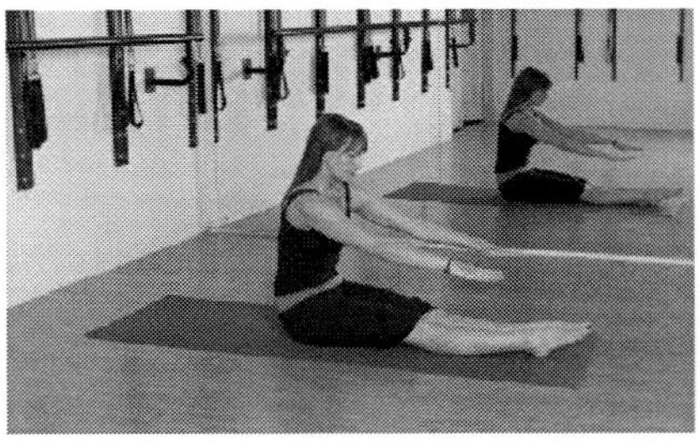

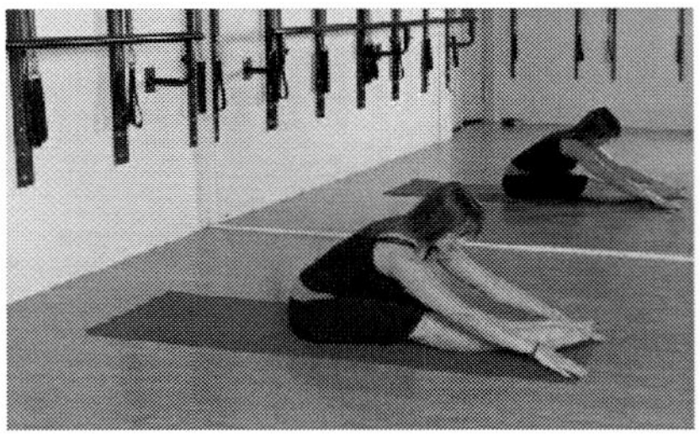

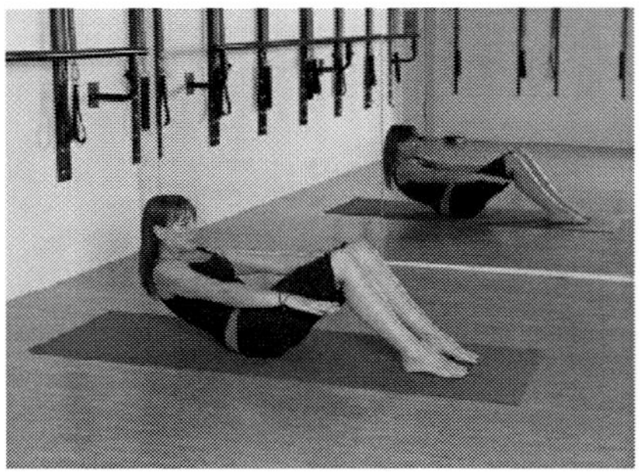

Variation Two

THE

STRETCHES

Spine Articulations
Hip Twist
Cat stretch
Thread needle stretch
Mermaid
Quadricep Stretch
Hamstring Stretch
Adductor Stretch against the wall
Hip Flexor/ Psoas Stretch
Glute/ Piriformis Stretch

Spine Articulations

Aim

To learn how to segmentally control and mobilise the spine, vertebra by vertebra. To stretch, release and lengthen the back muscles.

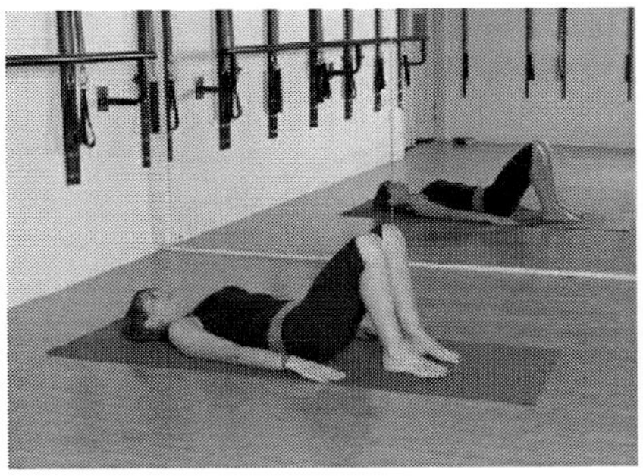

Starting Position

Lie supine on the floor in the relaxation position with the knees bent and the feet and knees are hip width apart. The arms are down by the sides of the body.

Action

Inhale - To prepare

Exhale - To engage the core abdominals and tilt the pelvis into a posterior tilt

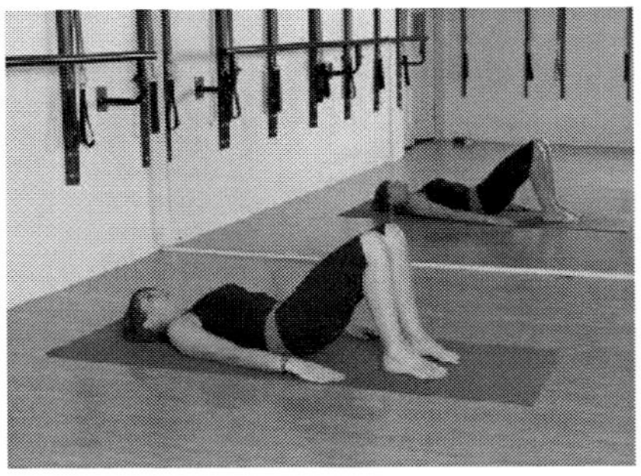

Inhale - To return to a neutral position of the pelvis. Start off with a pelvic tilt and gradually increase the range of movement as the number of repetitions increases if the spine becomes more flexible.

The breathing will change on the full spine curl as follows.

Inhale - To prepare

Exhale - To engage the core abdominals and gently peel the spine off the floor, one vertebra at a time

Inhale - At the end of the range of movement

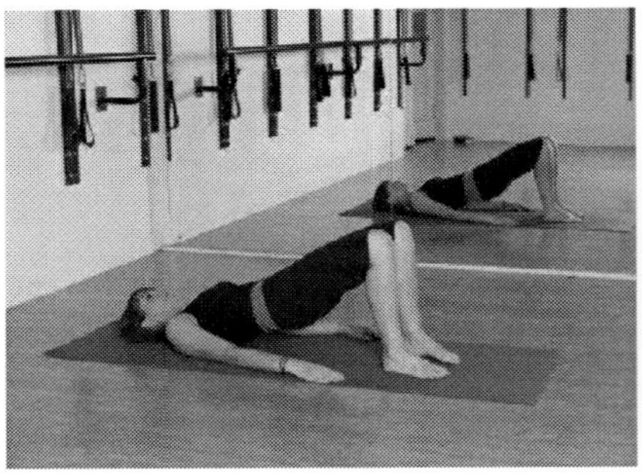

Exhale - To roll back down through the spine vertebra by vertebra back to the starting position.

Target Muscles

Core abdominals, hamstrings, gluteals

Watchpoints

- Ensure the back of the neck stays long and the shoulders stay away from the ears
- Try not to 'bridge' the spine by over extending the back
- Maintain good segmental control on the way down as well as on the way up to avoid moving the spine in one lump
- Ensure that the knees do not lose alignment with the hips on the descent

Variation One (Progression)

Add in the arms. Inhale to peel the spine of the floor, Exhale to raise the arms up to the ceiling and behind the head as close to the floor as possible. Inhale to prepare and exhale to return the spine to the floor, one vertebra at a time.

Variation Two (Progression)

Spine curls against the wall. This is the same as variation one except that the feet are placed on the wall (feet higher than the knees). The buttocks are a couple of inches away from the edge of the wall. Push the feet against the wall to provide extra resistance for the stretch.

Contra-Indications

This may be uncomfortable/unsuitable for certain disc related back problems

Hip Twist

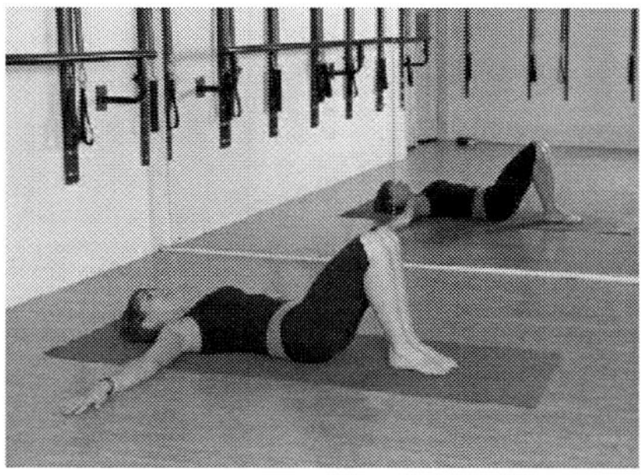

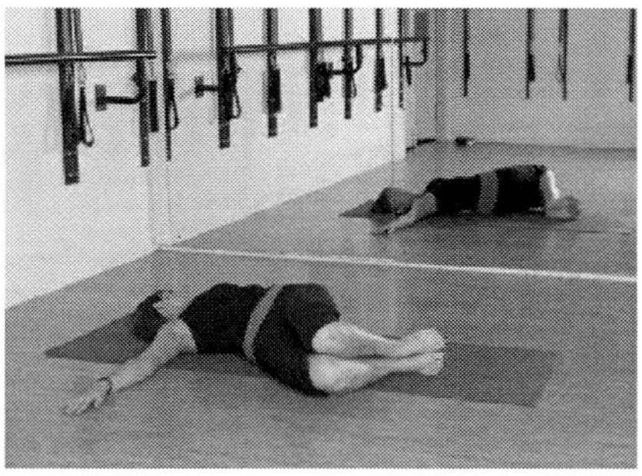

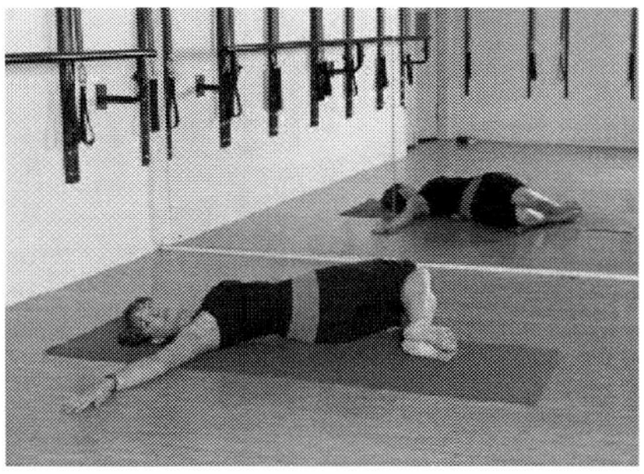

Aim

To stretch the back and neck and to open the chest and shoulders. Allow spinal rotation

Starting Position

Lie supine in the relaxation position with knees bent and feet on the floor. The legs, knees and feet are together. The arms are outstretched at shoulder height forming a letter "T" shape.

Action

Inhale - To prepare

Exhale – To engage the core abdominals and roll the knees to one side whilst the head moves in the opposite direction to the other side as far as feels comfortable

Inhale - Maintain engagement of the core abdominals

Exhale - To reverse the movement back to the starting position, bringing the head and legs back to the centre simultaneously.

Target Muscles

Core abdominals, anterior deltoid, pectorals, lats

Watchpoints

- Try to gauge the speed of the head and leg movement so that they arrive and return simultaneously (the head is usually only a small movement compared to the bigger leg movement therefore the movement of the head may be performed slightly slower)
- Ensure that both shoulders remain on the floor throughout so limit the range of movement if one shoulder starts to lift away from the floor
- Ensure the back of the neck stays long and the shoulders stay away from the ears
- Ensure that it is the abdominals (and not the legs themselves) that are employed to return the legs back to the starting position
- Only move as far as feels comfortable – do not force the rotation

Variation One (Progression One)

This exercise may be performed with the feet off the floor and the knees bent at 90 degrees above the hips to challenge the abdominals and stretch the back further

Variation Two (Progression Two)

This exercise may be performed with the feet off the floor with the legs straight and the feet are directly above the hips. The knees may be soft for those with tight hamstrings. This is a very challenging exercise. Whilst the flexibility of the spine may allow the legs to go further away from the body, you must ensure that there is sufficient abdominal strength to return the legs back to the starting position (if struggling, then bend the knees)

Contra-Indications

Rotation of the spine is not always suitable for certain disc-related back problems

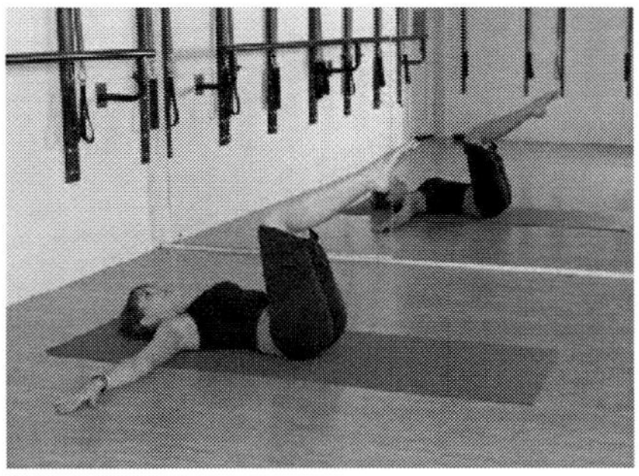

Variation One

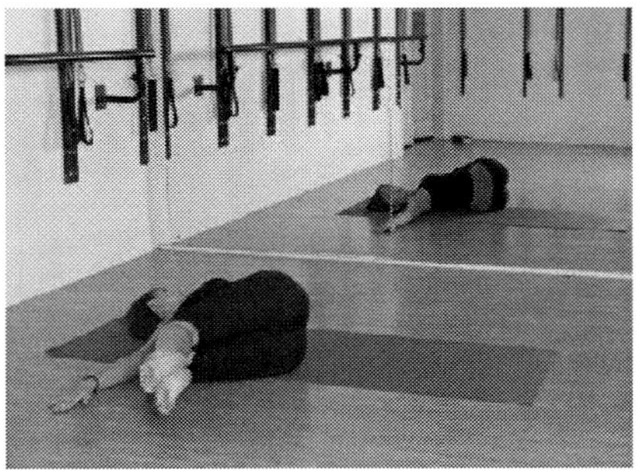

Variation One

Cat stretch

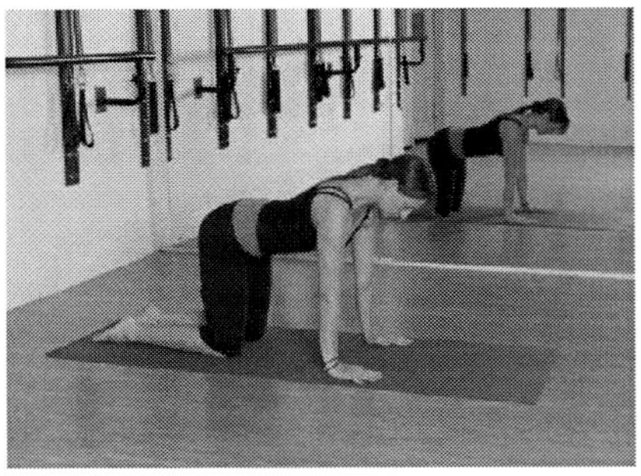

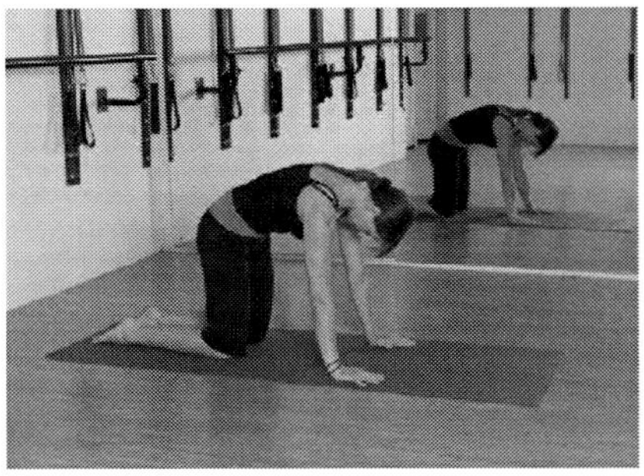

Aim

To stretch the back whilst learning to segmental control of the spine

Starting Position

Come to an all fours position with the knees bent directly under the hips and place the hands directly under the shoulders. The spine is in a neutral position.

Action

Inhale -To prepare

Exhale - To engage the core abdominals and tuck the pelvis into a posterior tilt and continue arching the back towards the ceiling ending with tucking the chin towards the chest so that the entire spine is in a flexed position

Inhale - To prepare

Exhale - To release the tailbone into a neutral position, allowing the rest of the spine to follow through, one vertebra at a time, until the entire spine is back in a neutral position.

Target Muscles

All spinal flexors and extensors

Watchpoints

- Ensure that the ears stay away from the shoulders when the spine is in a flexed position
- Try to ensure an even curve throughout the entire spine to avoid over flexing in the thoracic and cervical spine
- Maintain engagement of the core abdominals throughout
- Try not to lock the elbow joint
- Maintain an equal length on both sides of the waist

Variation One (Progression)

As for the normal version but instead of returning the spine to a neutral position, allow the spine to go into a slight extension, provided flexibility allows.

Contra-Indications

This exercise places extra stress on the knee and wrist joints and may prove unsuitable for clients with problems in those joints

Thread needle stretch

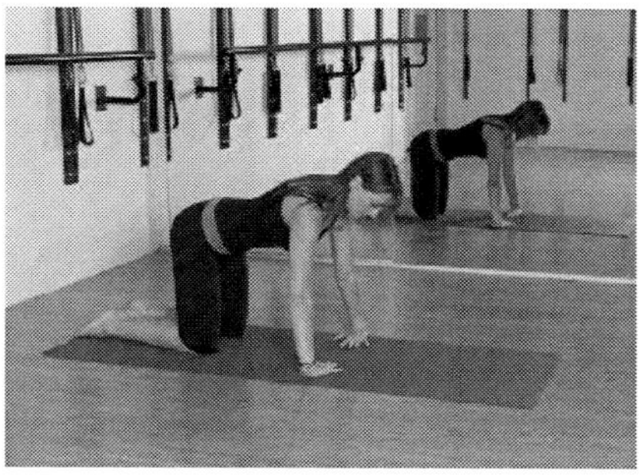

Aim

To stretch the back and shoulder muscles and rotate the thoracic and cervical spine

Starting Position

Come to an all fours position with the knees bent directly under the hips and the hands under the shoulders. The hands are turned inwards so that the fingers are pointing towards each other. The spine is in a neutral position

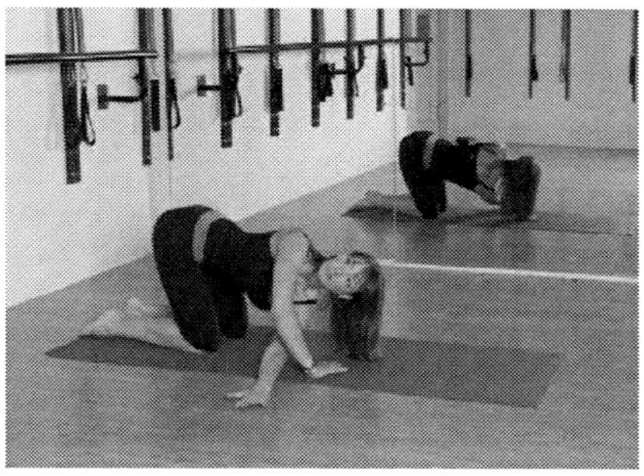

Action

Inhale - To prepare

Exhale - To engage the core abdominals and push the right arm through the body, passing underneath the left arm. The left elbow bends out to the left side. The spine will arch and rotate to the left simultaneously. The neck will be rotated to the left and the eyes looking towards the ceiling and the chest will be close to the floor with arm outstretched as far as the body allows and the palm facing downwards

Inhale - To return back to the starting position.

Target Muscles

All spinal and shoulder muscles

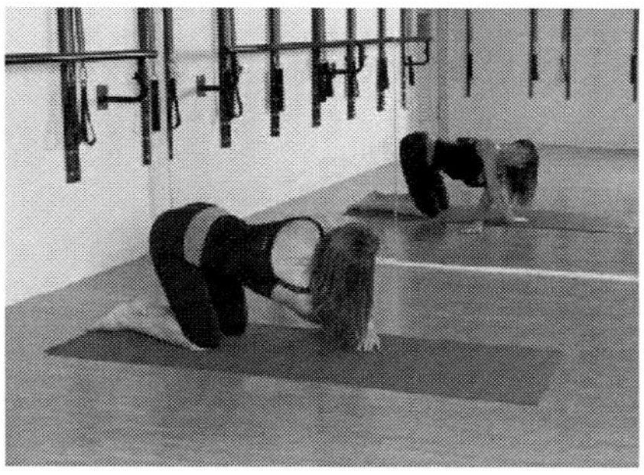

Watchpoints

- The head may be held in a more neutral position without rotating much (keep looking at the floor) for those with neck problems (or avoided altogether if turning the head proves a problem)
- Keep the shoulders away from the ear
- Maintain engagement of core abdominals throughout
- Do not allow the shoulder or head to touch the floor
- Maintain equal length on both sides of the waist

Contra-Indications

This exercise places extra stress on the wrist and knee joints and may prove unsuitable for clients with problems in these joints

Rotation of the spine is not always suitable for clients with certain disc-related back problems

Mermaid

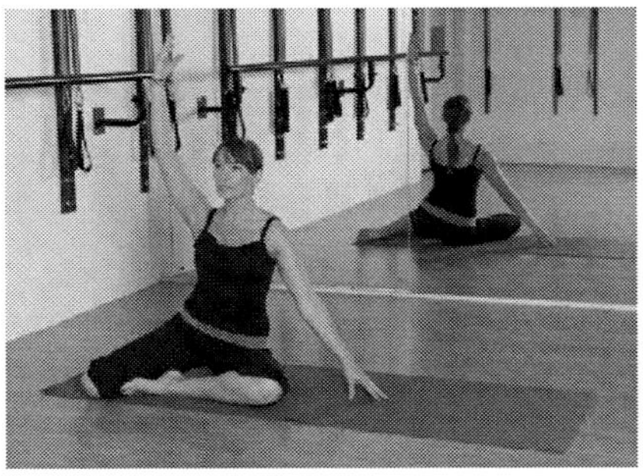

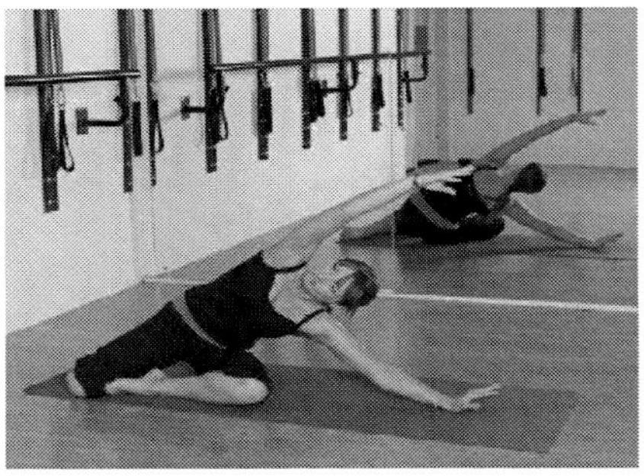

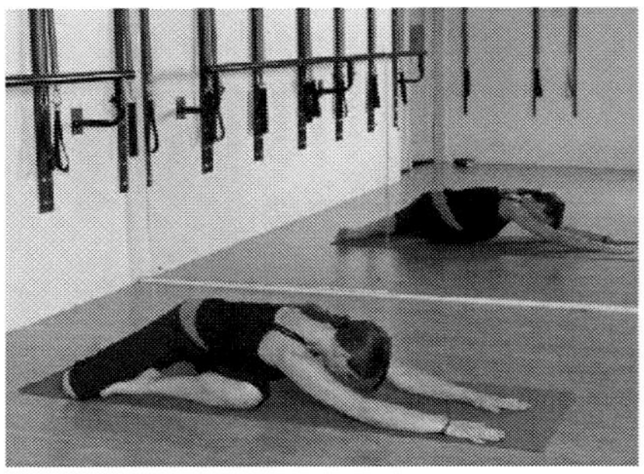

Aim

To stretch the lateral flexors of the spine

Starting Position

Sit upright with the knees bent on the floor facing towards the right hand side of the body. Place the right hand to the right side of the body and the left hand on the ankles

Action

Inhale – To engage the core abdominals and raise the left arm in the air above the left shoulder

Exhale – To stretch over to the right. The right arm stretches along the floor whilst the left arm rises up and overhead

Inhale – To twist the body towards the floor and place both hands on the floor and then push the hands further along the floor by a few inches. As you do this, the body will move closer to the floor

Exhale - To rotate the spine back again and then return to the starting position.

Target Muscles

Core abdominals, obliques, deltoids, latissimus dorsi, quadratus lumborum

Watchpoints

- Keep both shoulders level and away from the ears
- Maintain good oblique engagement to support the ribcage in order to prevent them from flaring
- Try to keep the waist long on both sides to prevent collapsing on one side
- Ensure the head does not poke forwards
- Ensure that the opposite hip does not lift too much in the side stretch. Resist the movement with this hip as the spine laterally flexes

Variation One (Progression)

This exercise may be performed with a side bend to the opposite direction. Start and finish the exercise as above. Then take the right hand off the floor and raise the right arm in the air. This time, perform a side bend to the left in the opposite direction.

Contra-Indications

For certain disc related back problems, spinal twists may be unsuitable. This exercise may be performed without the added twist.

Quadricep Stretch

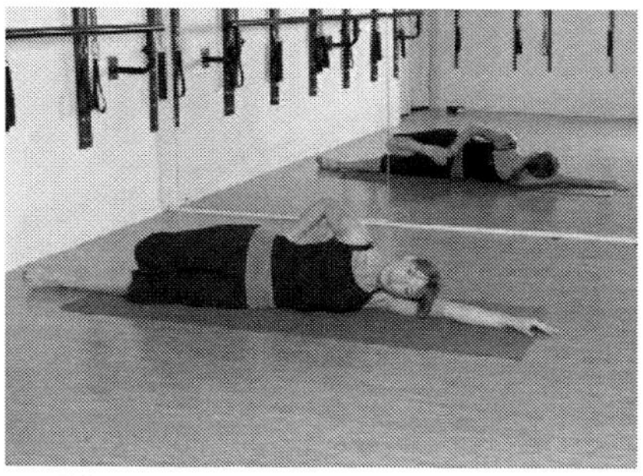

Aim

To stretch the quadriceps

Starting Position

Lie on the floor on the left hand side of the body. The knees are bent and the feet, knees and hips are stacked on top of each other. The knees are bent in front of the body at around 80 degrees (or wherever a neutral spine allows). The underneath arm is outstretched along the floor with the head resting on the shoulder.

Action

Inhale - To prepare

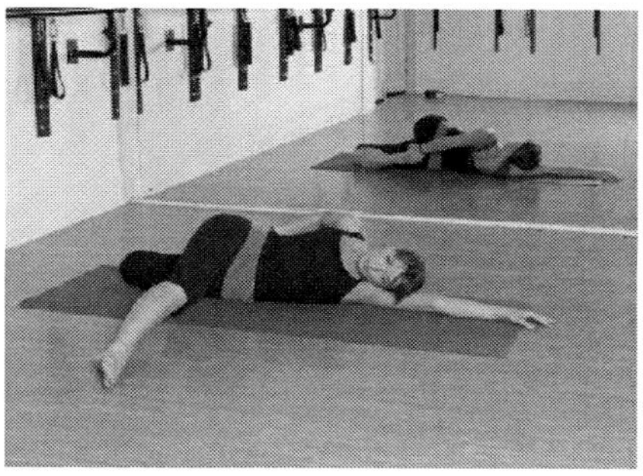

Exhale – To straighten the top leg forwards. With the top hand, take hold of the foot of the bottom leg and guide the thigh backwards and away from the front leg as far as possible in order to feel a stretch down the front of the thigh

Target Muscles

Quadriceps, hip flexors

Watchpoints

- Ensure the back of the neck stays long and the shoulders stay away from the ears
- Try to get the heel of the underneath leg to touch the buttocks
- As the bottom thigh pulls backwards, try not to let the top thigh move backwards

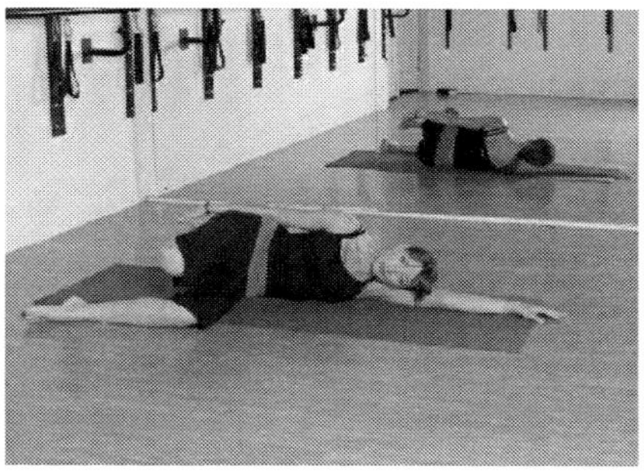

Variation One

Variation One (Progression)

Adopt the same starting position as above. Take hold of the top heel with the top arm and pull the top thigh backwards, keeping the heel as close to the buttocks as possible, whilst maintaining the position of the underneath leg.

Contra-Indications

The twisting action may be uncomfortable/unsuitable for certain disc related back problems

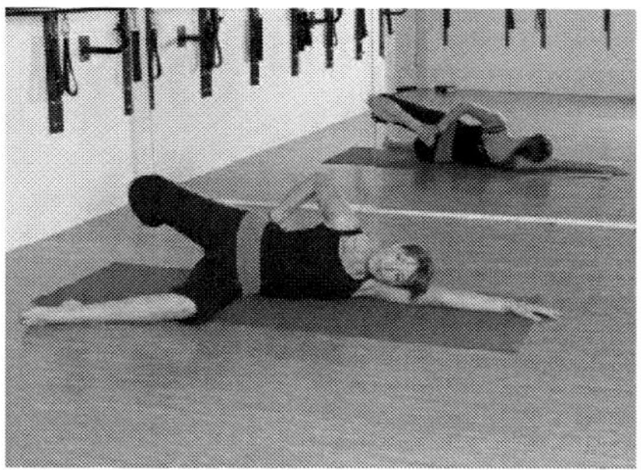

Variation One

Hamstring Stretch

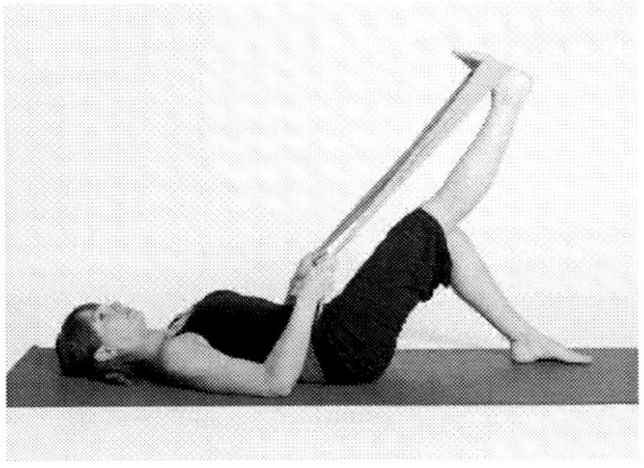

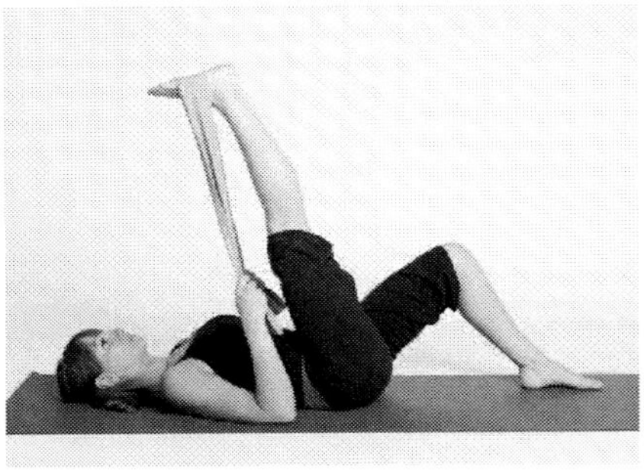

Aim

To stretch the hamstrings whilst maintaining a neutral pelvis

Starting Position

Lying supine on the floor with both knees bent. Bend one knee in towards the chest and place a stretch band behind the ball of the foot. The band is held in both hands with the elbows bent and elbows on the floor.

Action

Inhale - To straighten the bent leg away from the body

Exhale - Gently bring the leg towards the chest trying to keep it as straight as possible with the foot softly pointed. Continue bringing the leg as close to the body as a neutral pelvis allows.

Target Muscles

Hamstrings

Watchpoints

- Ensure that the tailbone remains in contact with the floor so that a neutral pelvis is maintained
- The waist should remain long and equal on both sides to avoid any hip hitching
- Keep shoulders relaxed away from the ears
- Ensure spine stays in neutral with the head on the floor
- Keep neck long

Variation One (Adaptation)

The knee may be kept bent as an alternative stretch for those with tight hamstrings so that the leg may come closer to the body and the pelvis still remain neutral

Variation Two (Progression)

The foot may flex in order to obtain a nerve stretch

Adductor Stretch against the wall with side bend

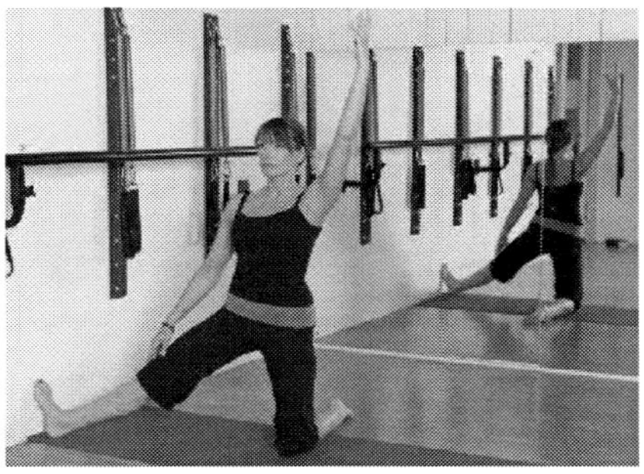

Aim

To stretch the adductors and lateral spinal flexors

Starting Position

Kneel upright on a mat next to a wall. Straighten the leg nearest to the wall and place the sole of the foot against the wall. The other knee remains bent.

Action

Inhale - To lengthen the arm furthest away from the wall up above the head

Exhale – To side bend over towards the wall. Hold for a minimum of 30 seconds breathing easily throughout.

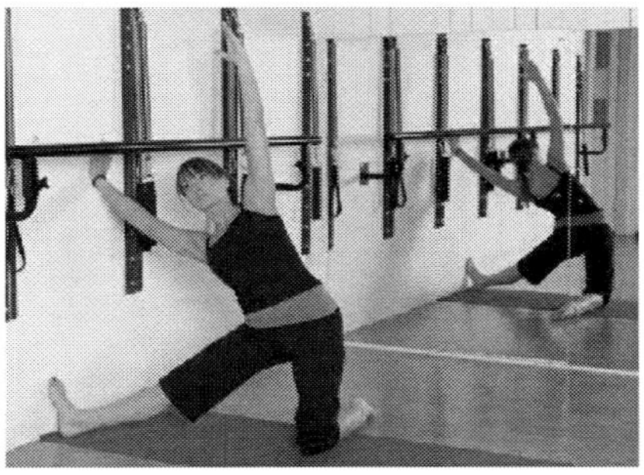

Target Muscles

Adductors, hamstrings

Watchpoints

- Keep neck long
- Try not to twist towards the wall
- Keep the pelvis as square as possible

Variation One (Progression)

Perform the standard stretch version but add in a spinal twist away from the wall, provided flexibility allows

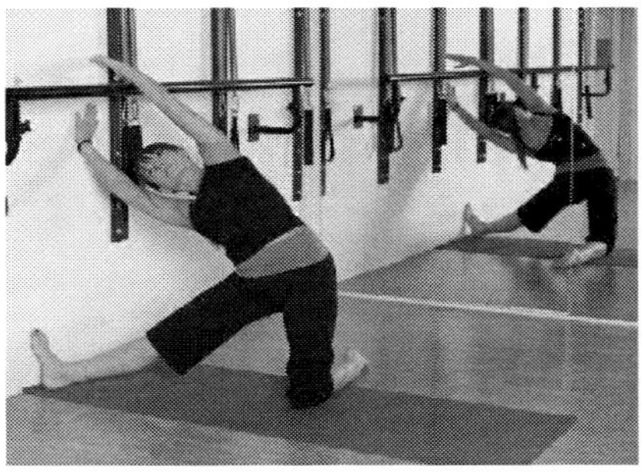

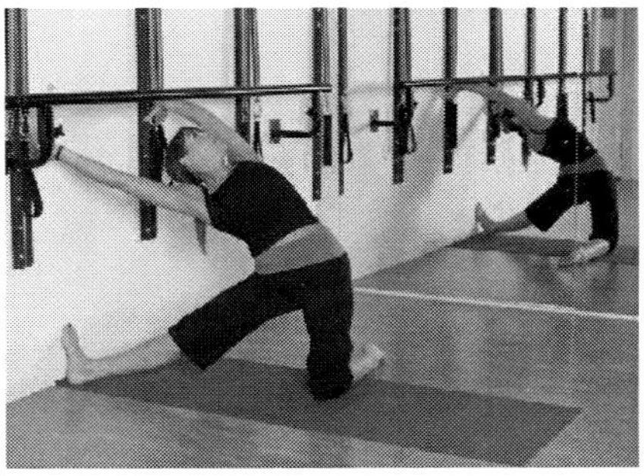

Variation One

Hip Flexor/ Psoas Stretch

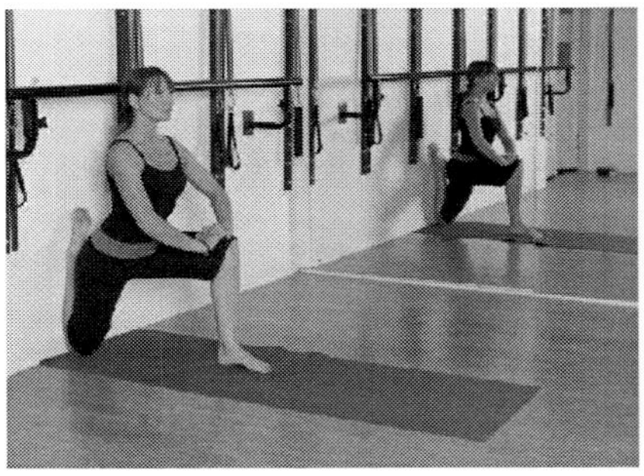

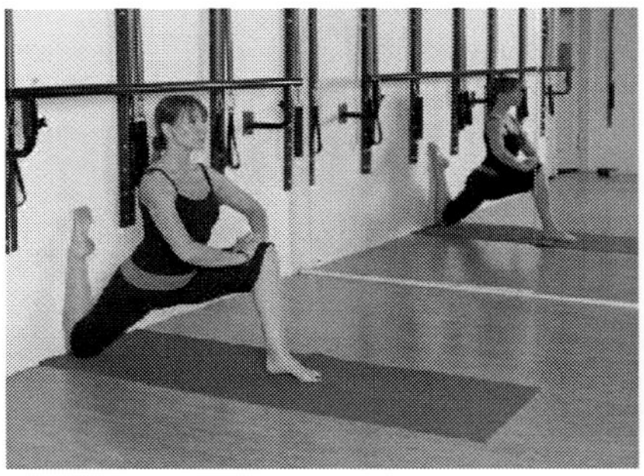

Aim

To stretch and open out the hip flexors

Starting Position

Kneel upright with your back against the wall. Place one knee on a cushion on the floor, as close to the wall as the body allows. The lower leg is bent backwards with the foot against the wall. Bring the other leg forwards so that the knee is bent at around 90 degrees with the foot flat on the floor.

Action

Inhale - To prepare

Exhale - To lunge forwards, increasing knee flexion on the front leg. Aim to push the pubic bone forwards towards the front heel.

For an extra stretch, perform a posterior pelvic tilt.

Target Muscles

Iliopsoas

Watchpoints

- Ensure that the ears stay away from the shoulders
- Maintain an equal length on both sides of the waist
- Try not to allow the front knee to move in front of the ankle

Variation One (Adaptation)

As above but the hands remain on the floor, either side of the feet. The less upright the torso is, the less stretch will be felt.

Variation Two (Adaptation)

Lie supine in the relaxation position. Slide the right leg away from the body until it is straight along the floor. Bend the left knee in towards the chest and hug it with the hands to achieve a basic hip flexor stretch on the right leg.

Contra-Indications

This exercise places extra stress on the knee joints and may prove unsuitable for clients with problems in these joints. Choose variation two instead.

Glute/ Piriformis Stretch

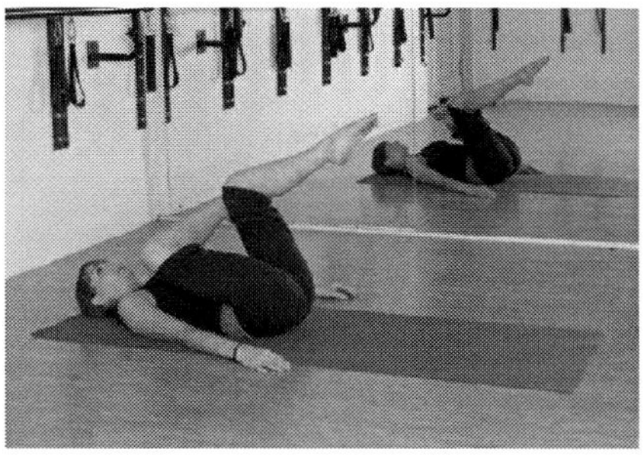

Aim

To stretch the gluteal muscles

Starting Position

Lying supine on the floor with both knees bent. Bend the right knee and cross the right ankle over the left thigh, turn the knee out to the side.

Action

Inhale – To prepare

Exhale - Take the left foot off the floor and bend the legs in towards the chest. Place the right hand in front of the right knee and encourage it to push outwards to the side. Place the left hand behind the left thigh and encourage the leg to pull inwards towards the chest.

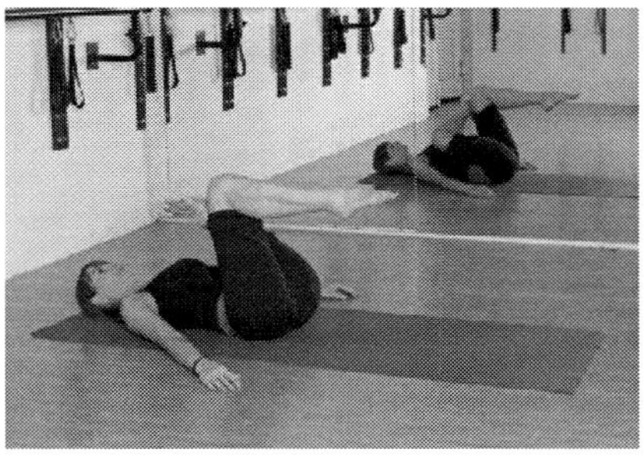

Target Muscles

Piriformis, glute medius and minimus

Watchpoints

- Try to keep the head on the floor or place enough cushions under the skull to encourage the head to stay on the floor
- The waist should remain long and equal on both sides to avoid any hip hitching
- Keep shoulders relaxed away from the ears
- Keep neck long

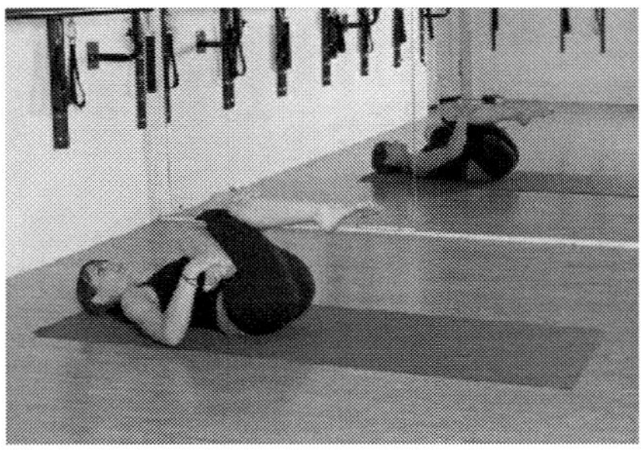

Variation One

Variation One (Adaptation)

Cross the right thigh over the left thigh so that there is no gap between the legs. Take both feet off the floor and bring the knees into the chest as far as possible. Place the left hand over the top of the right foot and bring the right heel down towards the left hip. Place the right hand over the top of the left knee and bring the knee further towards the chest.

Contra-Indications

If the turned out position of the knee is uncomfortable due to the twist involved then try the alternative stretch in variation one.

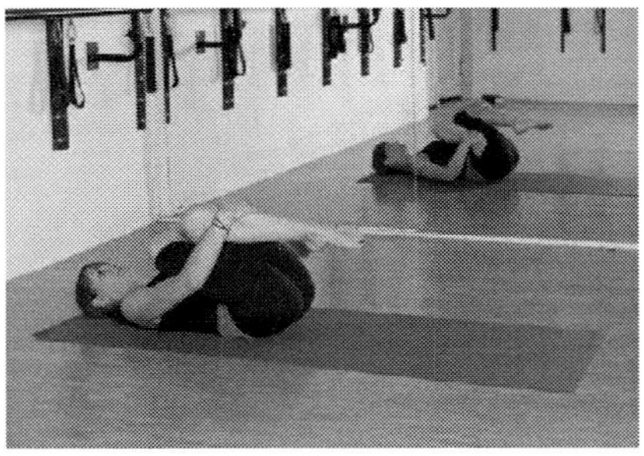

Variation One

Founder of Pilates Union, Emma Newham, has been in the fitness industry for over 15 years, teaching mind body holistic exercise including Pilates, yoga and **Gyrotonic** ®. She is author to 8 Pilates training manuals and has produced her own Pilates DVD's. Her company runs Pilates teacher training courses and workshops that are approved by The Register of Exercise Professionals. Emma has a wealth of media experience, having written for national newspapers and fitness magazines as well as hosting her live fitness shows on UK radio. Many top level international athletes including footballers, cricketers and dancers have worked with Emma to enhance their career. Emma presents internationally in many different countries, helping to spread the popularity of the Pilates experience. Emma also runs the highly successful, MyBody Studios in Northern England.

Current titles in Pilates Union: The Instruction Series are –

Beginners and Intermediate Reformer Manual
Comprehensive Matwork Manual
BarreConcept Manual
BarreConcept with Props Manual
Small Ball Workout
Foam Roller Challenge
Power Ring Workout
Stretch Band Challenge
Gymnastic Ball Workout

For more information on Pilates training courses or to order any manuals or DVD's in this series, visit www.pilatesunion.com